Methods of Childbirth

Methods of Childbirth

A Complete Guide to
Childbirth Classes and
Maternity Care

Constance A. Bean

618.2
B37m

1972
DOUBLEDAY & COMPANY, INC., GARDEN CITY, NEW YORK

To David and Carolyn
whose arrival meant so much to me
and inspired my continuing interest
in the ways childbirth is handled

Acknowledgments

I wish to thank the Boston Association for Childbirth Education, Inc. which has given opportunity for learning and sharing and which has offered its help so generously to so many couples. I am also indebted to the many couples who have shared their experiences. It is not possible to list all the people who have made contributions to childbirth education in the Boston area. In addition to those listed, other parents, instructors, hospital nurses, and doctors are working to improve childbirth and maternity care experiences.

Among those who have long been actively involved and who have known that prepared childbirth is workable and valuable are: Abigail Avery, R.N., Diane Bimbo, R.N., Joseph Bettencourt, M.D., T. Berry Brazelton, M.D., Max J. Bulian, M.D., Nancy Maloney Chandler, R.N., Gerald Cohen, M.D., Dan Ditmore, M.D., Karla Ellenbogen, Sumner Gochberg, M.D., Florence Hoff, R.N., Justine Kelliher, R.N., Barbara Krukonis, R.N., Sally Mack, M.S.W., Adelaide McGarrett, R.P.T., Susan Middleton, R.N., Mary O'Brien, R.N., Ronald Parker, M.D., John Reichard, M.D., G. Robert Rigsby, M.D., Barbara Roderick, R.N., Hilary Salk, Sylvia Sawin, Mary Shaw, R.N., David and Patricia Stone, Norma Swenson, Marion Tratnyek, R.N., Elizabeth Wallingford, Linda Wabrek, R.P.T.,

James Whelton, M.D., and Clement Yahia, M.D. The manuscript was read by Norma Swenson, Eve Hammer-schmidt, Dr. Bulian, and Dr. Yahia.

I wish to thank also the Ella Lyman Cabot Trust which helped to support a study of childbirth classes and the preparation of this book.

Additionally, I would like to thank Doubleday & Company, especially Lisa Drew, for giving such interest and detailed attention to the publishing of this book.

Contents

PREFACE

Education for childbirth began as a way of relieving pain in childbirth. It demonstrated physical and emotional benefits for the new family. Soon it was challenging pet theories and practices surrounding birth. It now offers couples some choices which will affect them and their babies very much.

This book will explain what goes on in the seemingly mysterious childbirth classes, what goes on in the woman's body during and after birth, and what happens during her hospital stay.

Although the available methods of preparation have more similarities than differences as they have developed, they do tend to create uncertainties among those who want to understand the techniques taught and why these techniques are so effective in relieving the pain of childbirth. Obstetricians and nurses, as well as expectant parents, ask questions about Lamaze childbirth, husbands in labor and delivery, and the rooming-in of mother and baby at the hospital.

When childbirth moved into the hospital women were tense and fearful among strangers. Medication could be given more easily in the hospital and it helped to relieve their fears. Progress in the development of anesthesia and the ability to resuscitate infants encouraged the removal of women from the birth experience even when the delivery was normal. Also, the suffragette movement of that era encouraged women desiring their freedom to wish to be liberated from childbirth. The rigid infant care practices of that time fitted in well with hospital routines.

Women today are beginning to ask for liberation from the dehumanizing aspects of maternity care which have acted to render them ignorant and helpless at the time of birth. Because possible problems have become more amenable to medical management, attention can turn to other needs of parents and babies. Their comfort can be seen as more important than adherence to rigid and out-dated routines.

The fields of obstetrics and childbirth education, though interdependent, are not the same. In general, the development of childbirth education came after that of obstetrics. It started with the discovery of "natural childbirth," which required that women be taught the exercises and breathing techniques needed to share in an awake and participating experience. Childbirth education received support from modern nurse-midwifery with its understanding of normal childbearing. It has developed as an interdisciplinary field in which relevant information from education, obstetrics, pediatrics, nursing, the social sciences, health education, physiology, physical therapy, and mental health has been synthesized into a practical program for parents. No longer is a prenatal class limited to diaper changing, baby baths, and formula making.

Because the demand for the new childbirth has come mostly from parents, the situation has often arisen that those parents who have learned about prepared childbirth often have more information available to them than do doctors and nurses or other workers involved in their care. Some doctors and nurses have learned about prepared childbirth on their own initiative because they wished to meet consumer demand and can see its benefits, or they have learned because they wanted the training for themselves as they became parents. Childbirth instructors have learned how to teach parents from other instructors, from the obstetricians and nurses who have been leaders in the new approach to childbirth, and from books written about either the Read or Lamaze methods or a modification of one of these two major approaches. Instructors also learn by coaching women in labor and through their own personal experiences in giving birth and becoming parents.

Although most of the leadership in childbirth education has come from lay groups, both lay and professional leadership have combined to find ways of improving the quality of the maternity experience for parents. The International Childbirth Education Association, Inc., was formed in 1960. Its purpose is to apply mental health and public health concepts to maternity care, the goal being to promote the health of newborns and to encourage more rewarding family relationships. The ICEA advocates no one method of preparation but teaches various modern approaches to childbirth. The American Society for Psychoprophylaxis in Obstetrics, Inc., was also formed in 1960 to promote the Lamaze method of childbirth.

The majority of women having babies today do not have preparation for childbirth because of lack of knowledge and because of the small number of trained professionals. The demand is greater among highly educated groups, but programs for low-income people and unwed mothers are starting to become available. As childbirth education gains recognition and as hospitals place higher priority on patient education as part of their services, the importance of guidelines for classes becomes evident whether classes are to be sponsored by parent groups, hospitals, or schools.

A small but determined group of couples wish to drop out of much of the medical care system and have their babies born at home. They seek out information on childbirth from the local childbirth education association and they may come to classes. They also search for a doctor to deliver them at home. Occasionally, but not often, they find one. If not, they may decide to go it alone for the birth and to use the hospital only if they get into difficulty. They do want medical care, but they want it on their terms. Obstetricians are expressing concern about these home deliveries because of possible medical problems.

There are reasons beyond those of parent desires for turning attention to new babies and the ways in which childbirth is handled. In the United States more babies still die than in most other developed countries. The U.S. usually hovers about sixteenth from the top of the list with Sweden and Holland vying for first place when the annual data are collected. In no state does the death rate approach the low rate of Sweden, not even in Utah, the state with the lowest infant death rate. If the figures from the U.S. ghetto areas are removed, the U.S. is still tenth from the top of the list. The Statistical Office of the United Nations reports that an infant born in the U.S. is more than four times as likely to die in the first day of life as an infant born in Japan. The Japanese statistics are verified by the Statistical Office. The additional deaths in the U.S. are caused mostly by birth injuries, postnatal asphyxia, and lung problems. The major difference between the two countries is the routine use of obstetrical medication in the United States as opposed to Japan.

The poor showing of the United States has often been explained in terms of methods of data collection, the ghetto areas, prematurity, poor nutrition, lack of prenatal care, and the need for more medical facilities. However, deprivation, birth defects, prematurity, and low birth weight are not unique to the U.S., and 40 to 60% of early infant deaths occur in full-term infants of birth weight over five and a half pounds. The slight differences in collecting data do not alter the statistics significantly. More information on infant mortality, with documentation, is available in the 1971 edition of the manual, *Implementing Family-Centered Maternity Care with a Central Nursery*,[1] published by the International Childbirth Education Association.

Deaths are not the only problem. Windle's[2] studies tell us that nearly half a million children with minimum neurological deficits are born each year. This figure might have been higher if the evaluations had been made earlier than the age of one year. The Collaborative Perinatal Program of the National Institute of Neurological Diseases and Blindness found 1.5% of all year-old infants in fourteen of the foremost medical institutions to have definite neurological abnormalities.

Dr. Karlis Adamsons[3] of Columbia University, discussing conventional care, describes the mother flat on her back, pushing her baby "uphill." He says that 25% of infants suffer some oxygen deficiency at birth. Three to 4% are severely afflicted by lack of oxygen and may develop cerebral palsy or other handicaps.

Dr. David Rutstein[4] of the Department of Preventive Medicine at Harvard University describes the importance of oxygen and says that a factor in oxygen deprivation is the too liberal use of drugs and anesthesia given to relieve pain. He also comments on the too liberal use of hormones given to induce or speed labor. These hormones increase the length and strength of labor contractions, producing the possibility of oxygen deprivation. He mentions, too, the possibility of harm from the unwise use of forceps.

Dr. Abraham Towbin,[5] neuropathologist at Harvard, estimates that three million Americans suffer from minimal brain dysfunction resulting in a reduction of the individual's potential, behavior disorders, learning defects, reading difficulty, hyperactivity, or unusual awkwardness. He associates this brain damage with birth. He has also written a paper[6] on injuries to the spinal cord and brain stem caused by excessive traction and flexion of the fetal vertebral column during delivery.

At present the use of monitoring equipment strapped onto, or inserted inside of, mothers in labor, whether or not they are high-risk patients, is being widely touted as a way of reducing infant morbidity and mortality. However, there are practices, especially associated with the United States which some people feel are contributing unnecessary stress on the baby and contributing to the high U.S. infant morbidity and mortality statistics, even though these practices have their uses. They are:

1. excessive preoccupation with *limiting weight gain* during pregnancy.[7]

2. "babies by appointment." *Elective inductions* are convenient but are associated with increased hazards for the baby even if rigid criteria for induction are used.[8]

3. hormonal *speeding of labor*, which is especially associated with a medicated labor. Medication may be a factor in slowing labor and require that hormonal stimulation be given. An unmedicated woman is likely to find the artificially augmented contractions uncomfortable and will therefore require medication which she would not have needed without this stimulation of labor. The monitoring equipment has been useful in demonstrating the amount of slowing of the baby's heart rate during prolonged, artificially stimulated contractions.

4. *flat-on-the-back position for labor*. The weight of the pregnant uterus on a major blood vessel places stress on the maternal circulation and may deprive the infant of life-giving blood. A change to the side position increases the output of the heart by as much as 20% and more.[9] The back position, maintained over a period of time, is associated with the use of medication.

5. *labor medications*.[10] There are several studies on this. Brazelton found a twenty-four-hour delay in the baby's weight gain, delayed sucking response, and abnormalities in electroencephalograms during the early days after birth as compared with babies whose mothers had not received medication during labor.

6. The *lithotomy position for delivery* instead of the semi-squatting, somewhat raised position used in many other countries. The flat position with legs up in stirrups adds stress to the delivery.

7. *rapid clamping of the cord* after delivery. This practice may affect expulsion of the placenta as well as depriving the infant of blood containing oxygen and iron.[11,12,13]

8. *delayed infant sucking and feeding opportunities* up to eight, twelve, or even twenty-four hours. This practice became associated with the use of obstetric medications.

9. *low incidence of breast feeding*, especially for the premature and high-risk babies who need it most. In contrast to countries with fewer infant deaths, little encouragement is given to low-income women to breast-feed their babies.

GLOSSARY

Adductor Muscle. The inner thigh muscle.

Amnesic. A medication causing temporary loss of memory.

Analgesic. A medication used during labor to raise the threshold for pain perception or to induce sleep.

Anesthetic. A substance introduced into the body, usually close to the time of delivery, to block sensation in a region of the body or to cause loss of consciousness.

Anterior. The forward, ventral, or belly surface of the body.

Apgar Score. A scale in which at one minute of age a baby is rated by observation on his pulse, respiration, muscle tone, reflex irritability, and color. The test may be repeated at five minutes and at thirty minutes of age.

Barbiturate. An analgesic medication inducing sleep.

Caudal Anesthesia. A regional anesthetic introduced into the caudal or sacral canal to block the conductivity of sensory nerves.

Cervix. The mouth of the uterus.

Childbirth Education. Includes factual information about the childbirth process and preparation for participation in the childbirth experience.

Colostrum. The yellowish substance produced by the breasts for the baby before the milk comes in.

Conduction Anesthesia. A regional block anesthesia such as epidural, caudal, spinal, saddle block, paracervical or pudendal anesthesia. It does not block consciousness but interferes with the conduction of sensory nerve impulses to the brain. The anesthetized region depends on where the anesthetic substance in injected.

Demerol (or *Meperidine*). A narcotic which raises the threshold for pain perception.

Diaphragm. The muscular-membranous partition separating the abdominal and thoracic cavities. It descends when air enters the lungs during an inspiration breath.

Dilatation. A term referring to the amount of opening (measured in fingers or centimeters) of the cervix which has occurred during the first stage of labor.

Effleurage. The gentle, rhythmical stroking of the abdomen, first used in France, which may be used during the contraction.

Emergency Childbirth. Childbirth without anesthesia, but also without understanding, training, or control by the woman.

Epidural. A conduction anesthesia introduced into the extradural space in the lower back.

Episiotomy. The incision made by the obstetrician just before delivery to enlarge the vaginal opening.

Family-Centered Maternity Care. Maternity care focused on the importance of family unity and closeness of husband, wife, and baby during the days surrounding birth according to the needs and choices of the couple. It may include the presence of the husband in labor, husband in delivery, and conscious participation of the woman with hospital support, assuming prior education of the couple about childbirth and breast feeding. It may include some type of rooming-in arrangement of mother and baby. It is patient-centered care and may include all or few of these practices according to the needs and choices of the couple.

First Stage of Labor. The stage when the cervix dilates and the baby remains in the uterus.

General Anesthesia. Inhalation gas anesthesia which removes consciousness and therefore removes pain sensations from all parts of the body.

Gluteal Muscles. The muscles in the buttocks.

Induction, Induced Labor. A labor started by puncture of the membranes around the baby or by giving an oxytoxic drug, or both.

Lamaze Method. A directive method of preparation for childbirth based on the work of Dr. Lamaze in France who adapted the Russian psychoprophylactic method to his practice. It was brought to the U.S. by Marjorie Karmel in 1959.

Let-down Reflex. A neurohormonal reflex in which the pituitary gland is stimulated, usually by the sucking of the baby, to secrete oxytocin. The milk sacs then tighten and squeeze milk down to the milk-collecting sinuses.

Lithotomy Position. The delivery position in which the mother lies flat on the table with her legs up in stirrups.

Medication. Analgesic drugs such as barbiturates, narcotics, and tranquilizers which act to relieve pain in the first stage of labor.

Monitrice. A monitress, or instructor, who guides or coaches a woman through labor and delivery, usually using a method previously rehearsed by the woman. The monitrice supplements the regular hospital nursing care and is hired by the patient. The use of the monitrice was first introduced in France for use with the Lamaze method.

"Natural Childbirth." The term first used to describe the approach of Grantly Dick-Read, and is a term which has aroused as many misconceptions as permissive parenthood. In the past it was used to describe a birth during which no medication or anesthesia was used, whether or not training and education were employed. To some it can imply a primitive kind of childbirth in which modern knowledge plays no part, or a rigid system of no obstetrical interference regardless of circumstances. At present the term "natural childbirth" is usually used to mean *prepared childbirth.*

Nembutol. A barbiturate which may be used during labor.

Nisentil. A short-acting synthetic narcotic used as a labor medication.

Occiput. The back part of the baby's head which first presents itself as it crowns just before delivery.

Oxytocin or *oxytocic substance.* The hormone which stimulates the uterus to contract, is involved in the let-down reflex during breast feeding and in other physiologic responses.

Paracervical. A local anesthesia given by inserting the needle through the vagina into the cervix during the dilatation stage of labor.

Parent Education. Education of parents at any point in their development as parents with or without the accompanying physical preparation and training for participation in childbirth or factual information about the processes and events of labor, delivery, and breast feeding.

Pelvic Floor. The area between the thighs and between the vagina and rectum.

Perinatal. The perinatal period in medical statistics is considered to begin with completion of 28 weeks gestation and to end 1 to 4 weeks after birth. Usually the 1 week figure is used.

Perineum. The pelvic floor and the associated structures occupying the pelvic outlet. It is bounded in front by the pubic symphysis, in back by the coccyx, and on the sides by the ischial tuberosities (the bones one sits on).

Pitocin. A trade name for an oxytocic substance.

Placental Transfusion. Process by which the baby is held lower than the mother's body to allow the remaining blood in the placenta to flow into the cord and into the baby before the cord is cut.

Posterior Position. Position of the baby's head in which the occiput, or back part of the head, is toward the mother's back instead of in the usual anterior position.

Postpartum. The period of time following the birth before the six-week medical checkup.

Prepared Childbirth, Participating Childbirth, Educated Childbirth, Cooperative Childbirth. These terms are used interchangeably, each giving emphasis to an important aspect of the approach. Medication may or may not be used according to individual need and is not defined by any maximum or minimum requirements, but by whether or not the woman knows how to cooperate. Patients awake under conduction anesthesia such as spinals or epidurals, but without preparation for childbirth, are not seen as having prepared childbirth.

Psychophysical. A word used to describe any approach to childbirth preparation which uses a combination of psychological and physical techniques to achieve greater comfort, relaxation, and concentration so as to permit participation in childbirth, whether or not analgesia or anesthesia is used.

Psychoprophylaxis. Literally meaning mind prevention, and, more liberally translated, prevention of pain. An active, directive psychological analgesia aimed at preventing pain and modifying the perception of pain. A physiological basis for its success is also recognized.

Pudendal Bloc(k). A regional or conduction anesthesia, which anesthetizes the vagina so that the woman does not feel the baby leave her body.

Read Method. An approach to childbirth first used by Grantly Dick-Read and based on an understanding of the body, muscular relaxation, breathing techniques, and emotional support.

Saddle Bloc(k). A conduction anesthesia which numbs the parts of the body which would touch a saddle. It is a "low spinal."

Seconal. A barbiturate.

Second Stage of Labor. The stage of labor following the stage during which the cervix dilates. During the second stage the baby moves down the birth canal.

Spinal Anesthesia. A regional anesthesia which temporarily blocks sensation from the lower part of the body and also the ability to move the legs.

Spontaneous Delivery. A delivery in which forceps are not used.

Tranquilizer. A drug (medication) used during the first stage of labor to relieve anxiety and to increase the effectiveness of other drugs such as the narcotics and barbiturates.

Transition. The last part of the first stage of labor during which the cervix dilates from 7 to 10 centimeters.

Vernix. The white, greasy substance which covers the baby's body at birth. It serves to protect his delicate skin and to facilitate the delivery.

INTRODUCTION

There has been a great deal of writing in the field of so-called "prepared," "natural," or "family-centered maternity care programs" in recent years. Mrs. Bean, however, is presenting in this book what I consider to be a most valuable compendium on the various methods of childbirth; from a discussion of the traditional "old-fashioned" methods in which patients have been and, in some areas, continue to be heavily medicated, to a complete, thorough, and thoughtful analysis of programs in which the patient is awake, cooperative, and deliriously and consciously happy about a childbirth experience.

As a practicing obstetrician, teacher, husband, and father, I have lived through the period of "unconscious" childbirth to the present period of "conscious" childbirth experience. It has been a concern of mine for a number of years now to indoctrinate in my patients and in my colleagues a spirit of greater personal involvement with young couples in the parenthood role. There is no doubt in my mind that the young couples of today are more intelligent and more knowledgeable than in previous years. People today are better informed through the various modern channels of communication from a local to an international level—and they are also receiving more and better education in all areas of life and society, in terms of the educational process itself. As a result, young couples are more mature, more interested, more concerned, not only about the physical needs of each other, but also about their emotional needs, one to the other. It is incumbent on the obstetrician and, for that matter, any physician, to accept this attitude and to engender a very positive relationship with our young couples in fostering and furthering a more meaningful family foundation. For too many years, now, the traditional medicated or "unconscious" approach to childbearing has been one of fear and ignorance, one of complete subjugation to the omnipotent physician. Young people today resent this, and rightly so. Young men and women want to share the experience of childbirth, not as an entity of disease, but as an entity of health. No longer are patients told that they are being treated for a condition of disease, but rather that they are cooperating in a venture of health and prevention of disease. As a result, patients feel better during pregnancy care, have what I consider to be shorter labors, more normal and less traumatic forceps births, and better and healthier babies. There is a return to breast feeding and a more normal relationship in the postpartum period.

Mrs. Bean discusses, in the greatest of detail, and I am happy for it, the class content and physical exercise techniques of the "prepared" childbirth programs. She spells out the satisfactions and physical experiences of the childbirth process in a meaningful and graphic fashion so that the reader can feel, or would like to feel, this personal involvement. The book expresses the changing attitudes of hospital administrators, the nursing hierarchy, and even young physicians in training, toward a family-centered maternity care program. Husbands may now share the birth experience in both the labor and the delivery room areas in many hospitals. State public health departments and departments of pediatrics have adopted more permissive roles also in this attitude—having fathers present physically, and in a supportive role in the labor and delivery areas, as well as being present on the postpartum floor participating in the "rooming-in" arrangement. There has been no increase in fetal or maternal morbidity in these programs, and this is well documented.

The childbirth experience is a great and wonderful one —especially when shared and intelligently managed.

There is nothing like the thrill at the sound of a baby's first cry!

Max J. Bulian, M.D.
Assistant Clinical Professor of Obstetrics
    and Gynecology, Harvard Medical School
Assistant Clinical Professor of Obstetrics
    and Gynecology, Tufts Medical School
Consultant in Maternal and Child Health,
    Massachusetts Department of Public Health

I

Childbirth and Childbirth Education

Attitudes and Knowledge

> "It was all fascinating and enjoyable and a most inter-
> esting process to watch and participate in—certainly
> the most exciting experience of our married lives to
> date—he [husband] was a great support the whole
> time. Dr. ——— was so impressed with his help during
> final predelivery time that he allowed him to watch
> through the glass window of the delivery room from
> the corridor. . . ."
>
> *(letter written to childbirth education instructor
> from a student)*

Attitudes associated with childbirth have contributed to
public and professional acceptance of traditional ways of
handling childbirth, ways which are increasingly being
questioned.

Novels and movies have frequently suggested the agony
of birth, but women who may have wondered as children
how babies got born have grown up and become mothers
without any real knowledge. If women have not felt entitled to know how babies are born, then certainly men

have felt even less entitled to this knowledge. In our culture there has been little visual experience of birth and little factual knowledge about birth processes other than in the most general way.

The word "childbirth," the experience of childbirth, and the visual portrayal of birth are all highly charged emotionally. The response of the majority of our American population is still one of avoidance, the assumption being that birth is at least unpleasant and that the less one thinks or knows about it the less unpleasant it is.

How did such an inherently interesting and universal experience get relegated to this position? The traditional taboos on the subject of birth have derived from several sources. One of these is, of course, its sexual associations. The increased openness now possible on the subject of sexuality appears to be a factor in allowing more dissemination of information on birth, including the national television showing of educational films on birth.

Other fears about childbirth are related to pain and to safety. The control of pain is essential if a woman is to have personal knowledge and awareness of the birth of her child. The concerns related to safety are felt on several levels and may be associated with childhood fears and fantasies which can include fears of damage to oneself or one's baby. Moreover, the transition to parenthood is one that is both desired and feared.

Safety has been an important consideration in the development of ways of handling birth. The most important factor in the growth of the specialty of obstetrics was that of assuring maternal safety. The development of ways of handling complications through the use of anesthesia, forceps, surgery, and other techniques was important but gradually tended to assign all births almost exclusively to the realm of medical events. Therefore, both the public and the professional have tended to view birth as an act not really performed by the woman, perhaps only partly performed by the woman's body, but actually requiring little from the mother other than her physical presence. This attitude has tended to ignore the childbirth in terms of an important life experience.

Feelings about birth in the public mind have seemed to vary between visualizing it as so complex that it can be accomplished only by the complicated maneuvers of the obstetrician and, apparently conversely, so simple that the baby might arrive in the car on the way to the hospital. Of course, there is an element of truth in both views.

Professional knowledge about normal childbirth has been incomplete in terms of helping women respond effectively to childbearing. The number of disciplines impinging on the totality of the birth experience is an important reason. The birth experience encompasses the physical and emotional aspects of pregnancy, labor, delivery, postpartum, breast feeding, the case of the newborn, and family adjustment. Not all medical schools still require the study of obstetrics. After medical school the obstetrical resident learns to handle problems rather than how to provide a beneficial experience for the new family. Later, even without training, he will be expected to be able to offer counseling in the entire realm of feminine events. An understanding of physiological methods of handling normal childbirth has not been encouraged. His job with normal patients, who constitute most of the admissions, is to order medications and deliver the baby. Teaching hospitals do research on techniques, such as monitoring and epidurals, which are tried out on patients in the hospital. The resident is required to demonstrate competency with these tools of modern obstetrical management.

In the past doctors and hospitals were not geared to provide the specialized knowledge needed by parents. Only recently have their prenatal classes begun to include information on birth, breast feeding, and parent-child relationships in addition to the information on pregnancy and the well-known bath and formula demonstrations. Information about childbirth is now beginning to be introduced also into an occasional sex education course. In terms of understanding the importance of the maternity experience to the new family, childbirth has been neglected, too, by most public health and mental health workers. Childbirth education leaders now feel that this information should be available at all levels in society as part of the preparation for adult life.

The source of the growing demand by the public for knowledge about childbirth can be traced to more than the increased acceptance of sexuality and the questioning of traditional roles and behavior. There is growing demand for consumer participation in all areas of life including education, medical care, politics, and environmental control. Furthermore, an increasing number of couples have discovered that a satisfying childbirth and early parenthood experience does not require that women be drugged, numbed or unconscious, and separated from their husbands and babies.

Many people have been surprised to realize how incredibly dehumanized childbirth has become, not only for the mother but for the baby as well, and certainly for the father. The dehumanization adds emotional stress to this important human experience and often even contributes to the physiological stress on mother and baby during their days in the hospital.

In the traditional care system there is no continuity of a caring person either during birth or during the days after birth. Many nurses, perhaps also internes and residents, see the mother during her hospital stay. She must form a new relationship with each one.

Although obstetrics stand alone as a medical specialty in which the mother-to-be is commonly called by her first name, the new mother cannot count routinely on her obstetrician being able to provide human presence, support, or understanding at the time of birth. Nor is the remainder of the care system geared to provide this. Although hospital personnel are present in the labor and delivery area, and on the postpartum floor after birth, the mother traditionally has been very much alone and uninformed as she accepts hospital procedures. The baby, too, is very much alone despite the nursery lights and the frequent noise from the crying babies surrounding him. Traditionally the husband has been kept ignorant about what is happening with his wife and baby, and separated from them. He comes as a visitor during visiting hours.

This dehumanization of maternity care did not occur because anyone planned it that way. Childbirth was moved into the hospital to increase the safety of mother and baby, especially the mother. Almost no healthy mothers today die in childbirth. Very rarely there is a death attributed to problems with anesthesia or some other unusual complication, but anesthesia also allows needed surgery to be done and it has therefore saved many lives which formerly would have been lost.

During the early years of hospital care attention to hygiene and public health standards which were then coming into being were very important in the hospitals, especially since antibiotics were not yet available to combat any outbreaks of infection.

The specialization of duties among hospital personnel came from the desire to have specially trained people in each aspect of the care. This plan had benefits but it did interfere with the continuity of care needed by most mothers and it also prevented nurses from becoming knowledgeable in a total kind of way about the mothers and babies assigned to them. Although the specialization of duties had a purpose, mothers have sometimes said that they felt as though they were on an assembly line.

If it seems surprising to find the charge of dehumanization aimed at the maternity sections of hospitals which are housing mothers and babies, one fact must be remembered. Hospitals were set up to care for sick patients. They are therefore likely to offer medicines, isolation, and very little patient choice. When healthy mothers and babies were moved into the hospital they needed instead human contact, nourishing food, education for childbirth, and help in learning to care for their babies. Of course, institutional care does easily tend to become impersonal and routinized, but for a long time this distinction between sick patients and healthy mothers and babies was not adequately made even though the length of the hospital stay for mothers and babies was decreased.

When couples learn about childbirth the opportunity is offered for changing attitudes of parents and of hospitals, parent fantasies about birth can be replaced with fact. Several years ago Dr. Robert Bradley[1] wrote a book for parents. He was among the first to compare the need for teaching women about birth with the need for teaching people to swim. This was a very apt comparison. The so-called "natural" responses to either the first or second stage of labor are usually not the most helpful ones, but women can learn effective responses.

Because childbirth is taught as a skill to be learned, one result is a very much reduced need for drugs during labor. For many, the need for an anesthetized delivery is eliminated. This result, of course, changes the birth experience from the parent point of view and also from the professional viewpoint. The woman has control over her mind and body.

> I felt much better this time than I did with the saddle block last time. It seems a shame to get to the most rewarding part and then be anesthetized. Expulsion was hard work, but not painful as long as I kept pushing. Once I thought a contraction was over and stopped pushing for a few seconds. It hurt until I pushed again.
>
> (*letter from prepared woman after delivery*)

Women should know about childbirth for reasons beyond those of reducing the need for drugs and anesthesia and the resulting physical benefits to themselves and their babies. Childbirth is not solely a medical event which takes place on a day henceforth to be known as the child's birthday. Learning about childbirth offers the opportunity to prepare for a new life experience with the additional opportunity to learn to understand and respect the functioning of the body. It also offers the chance to learn to understand and respond to the needs of the new baby.

There is also need for knowledge about breast feeding,

another emotionally charged concept. Breast feeding can be done in modern America without education in many cases, even despite the average woman's lack of contact with this process and despite hospital feeding schedules which are often still fairly rigid. She is likely to find, though, that if she does not have help uncertainties and avoidable difficulties may arise which will inhibit her ability to carry out her wish to breast-feed her baby.

Studies have shown that during the time of pregnancy and childbirth women are unusually receptive to the help of professional people with whom they come in contact. Attitudes toward birth and parenthood can be modified during this time of "emotional fluidity." A good class and hospital experience to help the transition to parenthood. If the husband also learns with his wife what is happening and how to cope, then he, too, can learn that childbirth does not have to be a fearful and unpleasant experience about which he should know as little as possible.

Learning about childbirth gives importance to childbearing. This may aid the next developmental step, that of child rearing.

The arrival of a baby into a family today is likely to be a rare happening. The need for limiting the size of families in the face of escalating world population increases the necessity of parent and professional efforts to make each baby's arrival a satisfying one for parents.

Childbirth Education

Letters such as the following come to those who work in childbirth education.

The Big Thing, and what I would not have done without you was to go without the spinal injection. I was really on the fence about it. Do you remember when I asked Dr. —— "What do you think?" and he answered, "There will be a great deal of rectal pressure and it will get worse." At that point I was all set for the spinal. But then you leaned over and said, "It's nearly time. The worst is over and you can do it" and so I did! You are right, the pushing stage does not hurt, although it is a tremendous urge. I believe I felt somehow weirdly important and essential. It is too bad that not all women are able to experience this participation because once I left the labor room and went to delivery I can honestly say it was painless.

Oh, I grunted and groaned some, but it was the work of hard labor meaning labor in the literal sense and not pain. What I shall never forget was the doctor saying, "Here comes the head" and this great sensation of the popping out of the head. Then didn't he say, "Give another push for the shoulders" and I felt them slip out—and then I saw the little blue feet and legs, and an instant later the whole perfect little critter. It was grand, and I felt elated. The whole world seemed wonderful. It seemed like my only complaint was that I had to stay on the delivery table for a while, and it was narrow and chilly, and I felt like sitting right up or standing so that I could see the baby better.

Gosh, I feel so grand! They gave me a sleeping pill, but I can't sleep. I just lie here like a nut smiling out the window and wondering how two deliveries could be so different. You know, the first was hell for me. And now this marvelous experience sets me in good stead and frame of mind for any future babies. There is some learning involved. I'm sure of that, and by gosh I'll have lots of confidence next time.

My thanks. . . .
> (*written to labor coach three hours after unmedicated delivery of second child—8 lb., 14 oz. She was sent to class by her doctor because of her first unhappy, untrained experience, during which she believed she received scopolamine*)

Preparation for childbirth is typically provided in a series of six or more two-hour class sessions. The instructor and her assistant work with ten to fifteen couples, giving information, offering opportunities for discussion, and teaching the exercises and breathing techniques for labor and delivery.

Nearly half of most sessions is spent with women stretched out on the floor on mats or blankets. The husbands are kneeling beside them to check their techniques and degree of muscular relaxation. They may be giving their wives a back rub. For this floor work the women have brought pillows which are placed to support various parts of their bodies as directed by the instructor. She and her assistant move among the couples to answer individual questions and to demonstrate with reassuring touch how the husband can help his wife to be more comfortable. The husband needs this training if he plans to be with her during labor and delivery. It is helpful and reassuring to him, and to his wife, even if he will not be with her.

There is a kind of fellowship within the group during the physical preparation. This seems to be as important as the benefits which come from the group discussion later on in the session. The woman is learning that she can control to a large extent the degree of pain which she will feel in labor. She is also receiving messages, directly or indirectly, from the instructor, her husband, and class members which say to her, "We care how you feel," and "It is all right to use your body in this way."

The physical preparation clearly has implications beyond coping with birth. The woman feels better, and she has less fatigue and backache during pregnancy. One of the exercises, the one for the pelvic floor, is directly related to sexual intercourse because it teaches the woman how to better control the muscles around the vagina and it increases the tone of these muscles. During the birth the ability to release these muscles aids the delivery. After the birth she again uses this exercise to tighten and firm the pelvic floor.

During a class the instructor might use a knitted uterus or charts to demonstrate what happens to the uterus during a contraction as it tips forward, its muscular action pulling open the mouth of the uterus, the cervix. The knitted uterus may be stuffed with a solid material or even a doll. The instructor uses it to demonstrate the muscular action of the uterus. The muscles are working to push the baby down and at the same time to open the cervix and pull it back over his head. The instructor might use another model to show how the baby's head slips through the dilated cervix into the vagina as if it were the neck of a turtleneck sweater. She will also show how the baby descends through the pelvis while explaining that the joints of the bony parts have been somewhat softened during pregnancy. The vagina has also enlarged to accommodate the baby. The students learn how the soft tissues give way before the descending head as, pushed by the forces above him, the baby makes his short journey down the birth canal into the world.

Knowing about birth processes makes it easier to understand the importance of the abdominal muscles and of controlling the activity of the diaphragm by doing certain kinds of breathing. Tension and anxiety from whatever cause can affect the functioning of both voluntary and involuntary muscles. Both are involved in childbirth.

At times some obstetricians have felt that parents should be given information on the obstetrical complications which may prevent parent participation in birth. Childbirth educators, however, feel that the medical problems belong entirely with the obstetrician. Caesarean sections, for example, are not described or shown in a film. Classes are designed to meet the educational needs of the woman anticipating the typical, uncomplicated delivery, needs which have been so long neglected in the interest of solving problems. Moreover, there is the futility of producing fears about childbirth when 95% of births are reported as normal.

If there should be a problem, the obstetrician may find that he can handle it better with a trained patient. She can respond to directives, avoid panic, and accept intervention such as anesthesia and forceps when these are required. Occasionally an expected Caesarean has been avoided because the trained woman was able to really relax and push properly.

Preparation for childbirth offers an added dimension to good obstetrical care. Its purpose is to help improve the quality of the childbirth experience for parents and to help them have whatever kind of experience they wish according to their individual situation and desires. It has become increasingly obvious that preparation for childbirth is important whatever the type of delivery planned and obstetricians are referring an increasing number of their patients to childbirth classes. Some class students come requesting "natural childbirth." Others come because they fear childbirth and wish a better understanding of it. Still others want information as they would before embarking on any new experience.

Whenever possible, it is desirable that hospital staff members reinforce what has been learned in class and be approving of the woman's desire for a conscious, participating experience if this is her request.

Childbirth education programs do not guarantee a painless or a drugless labor, nor can they, of course, guarantee no difficulties of any kind. Most women do not really care if they do have some pain, but if they have training and if they have the support of the doctor and hospital nurses with the father included if possible, an experience such as that described by a mother at the beginning of this chapter is very possible.

Since the result of education for childbirth allows, in most cases, the conscious participation of the woman, she is not helpless and unaware of what is happening. She does not play the role of sick patient who surrenders control of herself and her baby to others until her discharge from the hospital. She feels that having a baby is her business, too, and she wants to learn about herself and her baby. During the delivery she will be up on her elbows looking down between her knees. She is not going to wait until she gets home to become interested and involved in her new baby.

The new approach to childbirth results in more than a mother and baby "in good condition." It promotes the mother's confidence in the support of those around her as well as confidence in the functioning of her body. She takes a kind of satisfaction even in coping with contractions as she has been taught. For her delivery she is not flat on her back with hands strapped at her sides as the untrained woman usually is. Her baby can be delivered without the need of the nurse to push on her stomach, and forceps are not required routinely.

The fatigue characteristic of the untrained, medicated, and anesthetized woman is uncommon after a childbirth which has included emotional support and small amounts of medication used as needed. Frequently she is euphoric.

Parenthood does not begin with bills and interrupted sleep. If the new father is present at the delivery he, too, can share the drama of watching his child draw his first breath. The baby is more alert than babies whose mothers have received the usual amounts of medication.

The practice of delaying the first feeding of the baby until he "recovers" from the birth is often replaced by nursing him on the delivery table if the new mother requests that she be allowed to do this. This is still a new idea to many people, but the practice is occurring regularly in hospitals all over the country. The baby gets physical closeness and comfort and he gets some nourishment from the colostrum which is present before the milk comes in even though the amount he gets is small. Immediate nursing helps the uterus to shrink in size after the delivery and it reduces the amount of blood lost from the uterus. It also encourages the milk to come in earlier than it otherwise would. The mother herself gets food and drink, unlike mothers who have had drugs and anesthesia. These mothers may go many hours without food, therefore increasing their feelings of weakness and fatigue.

After a satisfying childbirth the mother may request hospital care which will allow her to keep the baby in her room for longer than the usual feeding times, either part of the day or, perhaps, all day. She feeds the baby when he is hungry instead of wondering whether he is crying in the nursery. Her husband can visit her and the baby, but the extended visiting hours and some of the routine interruptions are curtailed. Parents can get some confidence and learn to know their baby and at the same time have the help and support of hospital personnel.

> Rooming-in was delightful . . . my husband could enjoy the baby in the hospital, too, and I felt confident that I could care for the baby at home. . . .

At first the rooming-in of babies with their mothers resulted in great anxiety for hospital staffs. They felt that the mother was not yet strong enough and that the baby would not be "observed" adequately by the mother and nurses. Finally, they felt that the baby would be exposed to germs because the father would be coming into the mother's room. Even doctor-husbands had difficulty in gaining access to their own babies. Therefore, at first, babies who stayed in their mothers' rooms for longer than the usual feeding period were required to remain there throughout the hospital stay. They were ostracized from the central nursery.

Gradually the hysteria over family-centered care has decreased, especially since this type of care has been shown to be a protection against infection. The baby actually gets more exposure to infection in the central nursery than he does with his parents in the mother's room. Fathers who take the precautions of handwashing, masks, and gowns can be less of an infection hazard than the variety of hospital personnel who are in contact with many babies in the nursery. Also, hospital personnel are exposed to a variety of people, some of whom may be ill. At times they may even come to work when not feeling entirely up to par. If the mother, however, has her baby in her room, she sends her baby back to the nursery when she has visitors other than the father in her room just as women whose babies remain in the central nursery do not have their babies out for feeding during visiting hours.

There has been success in allowing the nurse to care for mother and baby as a unit. This plan provides sustained personal observation of mother and baby as well as an opportunity for helping new parents. It also reduces the number of staff people involved with each mother and baby, thereby reducing infection possibilities.

Erik Erikson, psychoanalyst and leading figure in child development, speaks about the new childbirth. He says in his classic book on child development, *Childhood and Society*,[2] that the opportunity to hear about the "technique of natural childbirth has been one of the most encouraging experiences of my professional life." His endorsement is unqualified. He comments on the relief of anxiety, the choices available to the mother, and the physiological advantages to mother and child. He refers to prepared childbirth as "a judicious mixture of eternally natural and progressively technical methods." He tells his readers that "the mother is able, if she so wishes, to watch in an overhead mirror her child's arrival into this world: nobody sees it before she does and nobody has to tell her what sex it is . . . the emotional impact of this unique experience and of the full reactivity to the clarion call of the baby's first cry arouses . . . a permeating sense of mutuality."

Conventional Childbirth

The traditional approach to childbirth has been very different from that offered by the prepared childbirth experience, but it is one to which women became accustomed. They rationalized its difficulties and requested it. The care seemed adequate, especially since there was no knowledge of alternatives.

The dehumanization came to be accepted, and even as desirable and normal. The surgical model was the model used for handling childbirth. It is sometimes stated that this concept seems to portray childbirth from the masculine viewpoint, or at least the stereotype of the masculine viewpoint. If this concept is used, the pain is supposedly taken care of by medication. Birth itself is of no interest to the parents and an unpleasant experience to know about or participate in. Parents can concern themselves with the child later. Efficiency is best served by compartmentalizing staff duties at the cost of continuity of care. Until relatively recently few complaints were made from the public, which lacked both knowledge and feelings of entitlement to choices about birth, the postpartum period, and early infant care. The traditional system therefore seemed workable for a long time.

The traditional ways of handling birth tended to separate families in a quite abitrary manner. The hospital care system provided no encouragement to play any voluntary role in the birth and little encouragement to show interest in the care of the baby. This has been true for both clinic and private patients. Most women have accepted this. Handling the birth in any other way has seemed too much like "natural" childbirth, and therefore painful, without the realization that there is anything missing in their experience which education could help.

Actually the conventional experience has a good deal of discomfort when considered in its totality. Women report that the time between admission and delivery can be lonely. There is often no real feeling of communication with anybody. The woman does not see her doctor for long intervals. She is glad to escape through drugs. She may awake to find doctor gone, baby born but gone, her husband gone, and herself in a recovery room. Although women are far more likely to be awake than formerly, many women still do not even know who was in the delivery room when their babies were born.

After the birth the new mother may have feelings of weakness and dizziness as she waits for her anesthesia to wear off, and is often surprised to find that she does not feel elated at becoming a mother. She may have no recollection of playing any role at all in the birth. She may have intermittent memories of labor, perhaps recalling the pain of early labor without knowing how to cope with it. If she saw women in the labor room who were delusional from drugs, her fear of childbirth may be increased. She also concludes that she was saved from a horrible experience only through drugs.

The baby is brought after a certain number of hours have elapsed, according to the administrative routine. The new mother is not sure how long this will be. If she asks to see her baby, the nurse's answer is often vague. The nurse does not mean to frustrate the new mother, but the nurse on the floor may not know, and she does not have the authority to get the baby from the nursery. The mother tells herself that she is too "tired" to see the baby and the nurses are too "busy." Sometimes visitors standing outside the nursery see the baby before the mother does. Somehow having a baby becomes a depersonalized, unemotional experience.

The woman, although prepared to receive her baby, does not really yet have a mothering role to play. She focuses instead on her postpartum discomforts. She may be bored and waits for visiting hours. She tries to rest despite hospital routines and the sounds of wailing infants each time the nursery door opens. She feeds the baby when he is brought to her, but she has no way of knowing whether or not the feeding satisfied him. She does not know much about him during his early days, nor does she know whom to ask. Should it be her obstetrician, the floor nurse, or the nursery nurse? Or should it be a pediatrician who has made a hospital visit?

The nursery nurses care for the baby, but it is hard for mothers to ask questions of them as they distribute the babies for feeding. By the time all of the babies are distributed it is time to start taking them back to the nursery. Since the nursery care usually does not include feeding babies, the nurses caring for babies cannot feed them according to their individual needs. Even the hospital records on the baby's physical condition and behavior during his first hours are sparse and minimal. The mother has little idea of how her baby is being cared for.

This traditional kind of maternity care, although seeming to have certain advantages, also has definite disadvantages for mother and baby. The depersonalized care would be harmful to the baby if it were continued, and it can, consciously or unconsciously, be seen as a model for baby care later on at home. An intense and eye-opening experience comes from reading a book such as *Child Care and the Growth of Love* by John Bowlby[3] about studies done on babies deprived of maternal care and the resulting "hospitalism" syndrome in infants and young children. The withdrawal of maternal care seems risky indeed when one learns that an institutional environment offering routine physical care without tenderness and relationship from a caring person produces physical symptoms and illness, even death, besides producing emotional withdrawal and mental illness! The symptoms produced depend on the baby, how long the emotional isolation continues, and how complete it is.

When mother and baby go home from the hospital the woman gets her baby, the laundry, and responsibility for the home all at once. This makes it harder for her to find pleasure in getting acquainted with her new baby. Neither she nor her husband knows why she often feels depressed after getting the baby they both wanted.

Getting a good start is important. How the woman feels about herself and her baby and how the husband feels does matter. Although some women like to abdicate responsibility for themselves and their babies in the hospital, others find the feelings of helplessness and lack of information uncomfortable and depressing.

Pain in Childbirth

Obstetricians have supported the goals of childbirth education programs which encourage education of the patient, avoidance of unnecessary medication, individualized care of mother and baby, and help with breast feeding. Why, then, have women often had such difficulty in obtaining the new kind of childbirth?

When women and doctors talk about preparing parents for childbirth there are certain questions which are most likely to arise. What about pain and the use of pain-killing drugs and anesthesia? What happens if women for some reason cannot have the kind of experience they have requested?

Women have long been intimidated about participating in childbirth because of the fear of pain. They may come to childbirth classes because they fear pain or the loss of self-control under drugs.

The control of pain is by no means the only purpose of education for childbirth, but it is a very immediate and observable one. The comment that the new childbirth requires either bravery or a high pain threshold is not heard nearly so often any more.

Labor is not one long crescendo of pain, culminating in the agony of birth. Women often ask how the labor contractions feel as compared with menstrual cramps. Although the childbirth techniques have been adapted for menstrual cramps,[4] there is an essential difference between the two. Cramps tend to come and stay. The essence of labor contractions is their intermittent character. They are wavelike with intervals between when the woman feels fine. They seldom last more than a minute. Soon after reaching their peak they start to subside. The contractions of labor are healthy and understandable: their purpose is to dilate the cervix.

Labor is sometimes compared with swimming in a stormy sea. Both require preparation to do well. Control, skill, and timing are involved. The mental image is that of meeting the waves and sliding over them instead of trying to run from them and being overcome by them.

Observers at labor and delivery cannot always evaluate the degree of pain or discomfort. The woman is concentrating on the relaxing and breathing techniques. She may be preoccupied with what is happening within her and be annoyed by outside interferences not directly related to promoting her comfort.

When discussing pain in childbirth it is necessary to differentiate between the first (dilatation) stage and the second (expulsion) stage. Most childbirth educators feel that women do have pain in varying degrees during the first stage of labor, even though occasional reports of painless labors are received. It is true that sometimes an unusually rapid rush to the delivery room has occurred because the progress was not only rapid, but there was no outward indication that she was not still in early labor. Other women have to work much harder with their techniques. Women find satisfaction in discovering that what they have been taught really does work. They also know that medication is available if they don't like what they are experiencing.

The same obstetrical picture is observed to represent quite a different experience for different women. Some have reported the nausea of pregnancy and the healing episiotomy as being the most painful part of having a baby. The support of those around her and the reassurance as to the normality of her progress are vital factors in how the woman experiences her sensations and how she copes with them. For example, she may be having difficulty coping with her contractions and feel discouraged. She may be thinking that she has a few or many hours of labor still to come. If informed that she is almost fully dilated, and that she will soon be moving to the delivery room, her whole demeanor can change remarkably. The previous inability to relax and to cope with the contractions seems to vanish.

The most difficult part of labor comes near the end of the first stage as the cervix dilates the last three centimeters out of the ten centimeters of total dilatation. It is called transition. Transition does not last longer than an hour and there is a space of time between contractions. It feels different from the preceding part of the labor. The contractions are about to change into the bearing-down kind of contractions of the second stage. They are frequent and intense. Although transition can be welcomed because birth is near, childbirth classes always give special attention to practical help in promoting comfort for transition. Occasionally a woman reports that she was not aware of transition and never used her transition techniques, but this experience is not common.

The assumption by the public and by professionals that the second stage of labor, which culminates in delivery, is the most painful part of childbirth is an error which has long been perpetuated, especially in the United States. The second stage, during which the baby moves down the birth canal, is described by childbirth educators and parents as not being painful in normal situations. This does not mean that there are no sensations during this stage. There is the desire to push. There may be feelings of pressure, perhaps feelings of stretching. Of course, the woman must learn how to handle this stage correctly. The unprepared woman who has an emergency delivery will most certainly be frightened, and she will feel pain as she tightens her muscles against the delivery without the benefit of the coaching given to the prepared mother.

The delivery itself would seem as though it ought to be painful, but it is seldom reported as being so. The pressure of the baby's head causes a degree of numbness in the birth area. The baby is wet and he has a coating of greasy vernix on his body which helps him to slip out into the world easily and quickly.

Medication and Anesthesia

The prepared woman is usually given control of how she wishes to experience the birth. Therefore, parents and professionals always want to know what childbirth education programs are teaching about drugs and anesthesia. A separate chapter is required to describe the content of what is taught but the approach used in teaching this material is important in understanding childbirth education.

Parents learn that drugs and anesthesia should be requested as needed for comfort unless the obstetrician feels that there is a medical reason requiring him to make the decision. Women are encouraged to have confidence in their own bodies and to learn well the relaxation and techniques for comfort which are taught, so that both they and their doctors can feel confident. Classes do not teach that medication or anesthesia will or will not be needed. This cannot be known ahead of time. For women who prefer a conscious participating experience, no instructor could express better the essence of childbirth education than a newly delivered mother who wrote on her delivery report:

> Conveying to the woman that she can remain in control of the event increases the likelihood that she will remain in control.

The element of patient choice in pharmacological aid is still controversial at times, and can even be seen as a rejection of medical care. At first, neither the obstetricians nor the nurses in labor and delivery were comfortable about taking care of awake patients who wanted "natural childbirth" or who had learned about childbirth and wanted to have some choices available to them. Women educated for childbirth are less likely to behave like surgical patients for whom only the outcome is the patient's concern. They are likely to feel an emotional involvement in all aspects of childbearing and, when taught the necessary skills, usually wish to control their own bodies during a normal birth. They may object to routine interference done for convenience, such as speeding of labor or the use of forceps, unless there is a medical reason.

Women cannot usually be left alone in labor without training, support, or medication. However, this does not mean that trained personnel are required to be present throughout the labor. This is a common misconception.

> Someone was nearly always with me when I was in labor, but during the few contractions when they were not in the same room with me, it was harder to relax and the contractions seemed harder.

Doctors unaccustomed to prepared patients have felt reassured if the patient is asleep, or at least has been given a drug so that she will not remember her labor. If the patient is not in control of her faculties, the doctor feels less need to be concerned about how she is feeling. Obstetricians can seldom remain with patients, although they keep informed on progress.

Nurses are responsible for carrying out the doctor's orders on medication. They have been overcoming their former feelings that it is somehow not right for a patient to be awake, to have her husband with her, and to request medication as she feels the need. As they become accustomed to prepared patients they do reassure women that drugs are available, but they avoid giving the impression that labor is not progressing normally and offer drugs in a way that gives the woman some choice.

The only drug that childbirth educators recommend that women not have is scopolamine. Scopolamine is still widely used for patients not prepared for childbirth, especially if they tell the obstetrician that they wish to sleep and to know nothing about the birth. Occasionally a woman who does want to know about the birth of her child will receive it if she has not been in good communication with her doctor. There are parts of the country where it is not used. A few hospitals are just beginning to act to limit its use, but many women are still being given this drug although some spokesmen prefer to play down its prevalence. Hopefully its use will decline as more couples prepare themselves for childbirth. Some doctors have never used it, but prepared women have to know about it so that they will not be frightened if they see other women under its influence.

It is not an analgesic and therefore does not relieve pain, although it is usually used in combination with an analgesic drug which does act to relieve pain. It removes memory temporarily and typically it acts to cause hallucinations. Its chemical composition is similar to that of LSD.

Nobody knows its future psychological hazards, but a woman's behavior during labor under its influence is reminiscent of a disturbed ward of an outdated mental hospital. Besides not relieving pain, the scopolamine itself can even act to cause increased pain and fatigue because of the agitated behavior and inability to cope rationally with the contractions. Patients are usually restrained in their beds in some way to prevent them from hurting themselves as they struggle under its influence. The awake mother, educated for childbirth, may get little attention while nurses are holding down a "scoped" woman who is trying to get out of bed. The "scoped" woman may think she is being attacked, she may be picking unseen things out of the air, crying for her mother, or withdrawn into a stupor. The unpredictable results are one of the hazards of this drug. An ordinarily quiet woman may behave in a very unrestrained way. Sometimes later she will have partial memory of herself under the influence of this drug and be embarrassed by what she remembers saying and doing, but she does not know that the drug causing such behavior does not relieve pain.

The drug itself acts to alter thought processes. It would do so even if she were not in labor. Occasionally she can be reached by reassuring physical and verbal contact on the part of the nurses, but nurses do not like to work with "scoped" patients. Many nurses have not wished to work in labor rooms because of the atmosphere there. The use of the drug makes it difficult to give anything but a custodial type of care and makes it difficult to treat women as competent human beings. Most nurses do not want scopolamine for themselves when they have babies, but for a long time many of them accepted it as a necessary evil for women frightened of childbirth. Some Europeans and Asians who have visited American hospitals have at first expressed surprise at seeing these irrational patients and been told that "Americans want it this way."

One of the most unfortunate results of the use of scopolamine has been that many women have not received enough pain medication because it is hard to tell whether the woman's protests are due to hallucinations or to pain. The need for pain medication is often ignored because she is not responsible for her behavior.

Scopolamine is still used because it does not pass through the placenta to affect the baby as do the drugs given for pain. The use of scopolamine allows a reduction in the amounts of narcotics and barbiturates used which do affect the baby. The "scoped" woman does not have to be heavily drugged with pain medication and, in fact, can be very much awake under light medication, yet later on she will not remember labor, however unpleasant it may have been. For this reason there are those to whom the use of this drug still makes sense, especially women who tell their doctors that they wish to "sleep" and not remember the labor. The doctor does not receive complaints about the labor and the patient remembers little or nothing as she requested. Therefore the drug seems to solve something for both patient and doctor.

Women educated for childbirth feel very differently. They do not want to go through a painful and traumatic experience even if they don't remember it afterward.

Medication varies in its effectiveness depending partly on how tense and anxious the mother is. The more tense she is the more medication is needed to relieve pain.

During labor the woman needs to know how the drugs may make her feel and at what stages they can be most useful. Because both women and hospital staffs are now more knowledgeable about prepared childbirth it happens less often now that a woman asks for something to take the edge off the contractions and then wakes perhaps two hours after the delivery.

Parent questions are illustrated by this husband's comments.

> You want drugs available, but not to be used to interfere with your training and techniques so you can't think straight. The doctor may think you are awake when you can't even focus your eyes, but his version of awake may not be yours. What is a small dose of something? How long before it takes effect? Will the nurse tell you? How do you know when you've had enough to take the edge off? You may think it didn't work so you take more, then suddenly you're zonked.

The authors of a recent obstetric text suggest that the prospective mother be familiarized with the broad aspects of modern obstetrical analgesia-anesthesia.[5] Flowers[6] has also written a book on analgesia and anesthesia which parents as well as professionals might like to read.

Analgesia is the medication used during labor either to raise the threshold of pain or to induce sleep. *Anesthesia* either blocks sensation, causing numbness, or it blocks consciousness, causing sleep. Most anesthesias are given near the time of delivery. The inhalation gas anesthesias are used less often now than the spinals, saddle blocks, epidurals, and others. Parents and childbirth educators also describe a natural kind of anesthesia which is caused by the gradual descent of the baby's head. The perineum becomes temporarily numb. This prevents many women from feeling the baby leave their bodies. They are surprised when they see the baby already delivered if they have not been watching the delivery.

Many prepared women hope to deliver without anesthesia even if they have had medication earlier in labor. This is a satisfying stage for the woman. She wishes to follow her urge to bear down to push her baby out. Most women can do this, but there is some controversy among doctors concerning the desirability of allowing these spontaneous deliveries. This issue has been frequently discussed, often with misunderstandings. Without experience in childbirth it is difficult to understand completely at first.

A spontaneous delivery is one in which forceps are not used. The baby arrives because of the muscular action of the uterus and the voluntary pushing of the mother. Prepared women usually prefer the spontaneous delivery. When they request a spontaneous delivery this does not mean that they want an untrained delivery such as might occur during an emergency delivery in which there might be overstretched or torn tissues and the baby ejected with insensitive force. Deliveries conducted under heavy medication and general anesthesia also sometimes result in overstretched or torn tissues requiring repair work. The use of spinal or other anesthesia to prevent a spontaneous delivery relaxes the tissues and interferes with voluntary pushing. Therefore the baby is usually removed by forceps. The delivery may be called an "outlet forceps" delivery and, in most cases, requires very little traction to remove the baby. The spinal-forceps delivery is useful when the pushing stage is prolonged for some reason or when there is inadequate relaxation of the vaginal muscles.

The use of the epidural to replace spinal anesthesia is becoming more common, especially in larger hospitals. The epidural also interferes with normal body functioning and, unlike the spinal, requires that a small catheter remain in the woman's back so that an anesthetic substance can be fed into it at intervals. The epidural can be given earlier than the spinal and is especially useful for untrained women, but trained women seldom care to undergo this procedure unnecessarily.

Although doctors know that trained women like the un-anesthetized delivery, that they feel better after delivery and even have less blood loss if not anesthetized, some doctors still have concern about overstretched tissues or pushing the baby against unrelaxed tissues. The doctor must be reassured that the woman has been carefully trained and can stop pushing when told. The doctor must remember to tell her when to stop pushing. He must also realize that women can release muscles in the birth area, including those which are deep inside the vagina. Most prepared women do well with spontaneous deliveries.

This issue seems complicated, but it will become clearer to readers as the discussion of prepared childbirth continues. Each woman must discuss her feelings and her training with her obstetrician. Some women like the passive-observer role offered by the spinal-forceps delivery. Others do not like conduction anesthesia of any type. Conduction anesthetics are regional anesthetics in which an injected substance acts to block nerve impulses to the brain.

There are obstetricians who prefer spontaneous deliveries for trained women unless there is some reason for intervention. Other doctors prefer the spinal-forceps deliveries and do them almost routinely. Most of the latter group will allow the woman to try a few pushes without anesthesia to see how she does. If a doctor does use spinal-forceps or other conduction-type anesthesia routinely, women like to know this. Otherwise they may feel that something was wrong with their bodies or their training, or they may feel that their wishes were disregarded. The handling of birth may seem to be more a medical decision than one to be decided by the woman, but in most cases her training makes a difference in how the birth is handled. Women do care how the birth is handled just as they care how the labor is handled.

Evaluation of Childbirth Education

The fear of the effect of so-called failure on the woman has occasionally been used as a reason for not offering preparation for childbirth. It may come as a surprise to some that women might be seen as "failing" in childbirth, that the word "failure" could be used in this connection.

Despite the often-repeated statement that prepared childbirth is not defined in terms of amounts of medication required, medical personnel do need a way of evaluating the experience and whether or not prepared childbirth is workable. Quite naturally they tend to evaluate it in terms of the amounts of medication required. Success and failure are the words used in our vocabulary when doing evaluations.

Childbirth, of course, results in a baby in any case. The fear is that, although childbirth preparation usually results in an experience which parents call a "wow experience," the woman might find herself playing little or no conscious role. Suppose she finds the experience painful and cannot use the techniques to control the pain? Suppose a problem requires intervention in the form of anesthesia, forceps, or a Caesarean?

Our baby was delivered by Caesarean section, however, we feel that the BACE classes helped us tre-

mendously. We were psychologically well prepared. . . .

Parents are told that success for parents is defined in terms of their satisfaction with the experience, not in terms of amount of medication, the presence of the husband, or any standard other than their satisfaction. If the woman feels pain and needs medication she should have it. She should have whatever she needs to improve the experience for her whether it be drugs or knowledge of techniques on how to help herself. She can participate to the degree she wishes or comfortably can. There is never a disadvantage in receiving education for a new experience.

Childbirth educators see the role of professionals as that of helping parents to achieve their desires by using a problem-solving approach instead of wondering whether the labor will progress according to some standard. This same approach is useful in breast feeding. Instead of being overly protective and denying the woman the opportunity to breast-feed just because some women have difficulty, or leaving her without assistance, which often has the same effect, she needs to be given the information which will help her nurse her baby.

If the woman who wishes a conscious and participating birth does not have this experience, she may well feel disappointment. Obviously, she wants a desired experience, but the disappointment will not be excessive if she does not feel that she was deprived of the experience because nobody cared or because the professionals in whom she had placed her confidence did not help her. If her wishes seemed to carry no weight and she was given drugs or anesthesia instead of physical and emotional support, she may be very frustrated and angry.

Fathers in the Delivery Room

Prepared childbirth has become associated with the practice of having fathers in the delivery room. If the wife is awake and relatively comfortable, the child's arrival is a life experience which she wishes to share with her husband.

> Birth was for me truly a moving experience. It was wonderful to be able to share this miracle with my wife. . . .

There are still many people who become upset at the idea of fathers in the delivery room. When the uninitiated visualize fathers in the delivery room, their feelings about birth, sex, and surgery all seem to converge. Love and the arrival of the new child tend to get lost. There are fears that the husband will not be able to stand this stress, that he will faint, that he will feel revulsion. There are fears that he will get in the way of those who belong in the delivery room, that he will be exposed to suffering and will be useless to his wife. He might bring in infection. The whole experience is just too "physical" for him.

The results have not borne out these fears. Men have not reacted this way. It would be difficult to find a prepared husband who has been in the delivery room and who feels in any way other than that he has been privileged to share in something rare and wonderful with his wife. Documentation of 45,000 husbands in the delivery room prepared as a legal brief in California[7] allayed many anxieties concerning this practice so that it is now becoming more available to expectant couples. None of the California husbands fainted, or got in the way of hospital personnel, or expressed dissatisfaction with the experience. None brought legal action against the hospital, a possibility which has concerned hospitals. G 1686964

Undoubtedly husbands might find a traditional labor and delivery disturbing if their wives were frightened, heavily drugged, or unconscious. Having husbands present has sometimes appeared to encourage upgrading of labor-room facilities and to promote a better atmosphere in labor and delivery areas of hospitals.

> I was happy to have my husband with me in labor, only wish he, too, could have shared the joy and delight of the birth. He was a great source of encouragement, helping me by wetting my lips, supporting my back, rubbing my back with powder, waking me up if I slept too soundly and propping my legs in pushing stage.

> My husband was extremely pleased with our experiences in labor. He was somewhat surprised at how effective the breathing techniques proved to be. He plans to be with me when we do it again.

Most obstetricians and leaders of childbirth education programs feel that if the husband thinks he might like to be with his wife he should receive the preparation which his wife receives. Obstetrician, husband, and wife must be in agreement that he be included. In addition, he agrees to remain in the place in the delivery room allocated to him at the head of the table and to leave the delivery room without question if the obstetrician asks him to do so. Some hospitals require that he sign some type of waiver or release before going into the delivery room. He is masked and gowned in the same way as others in the delivery room. Occasionally he is not masked, the reasoning being that if the wife is not masked why should the husband be?

Earlier, during the labor, he helps to remind his wife about techniques and provides the companionship which often may not be available from busy nurses. He often brings a sandwich so that he will not find himself going for several hours without food because he doesn't want to leave his wife. If he didn't eat he might then very well feel faint by the time the baby arrived.

The result of including the husband and new father is that he is less likely to have the traditional feelings of ignorance, isolation, and resentment of his wife's changing role. He also does not have the guilt so often attributed to husbands who get their wives pregnant and then blame themselves because their wives have to go through childbirth.

> The thrill of my husband as he heard the baby's first cry (he was in a hall adjacent to the delivery room) was important to the total experience because it has become an unforgettable moment in his life. I cannot find words to convey all that is in our hearts now, they are much too full.
>
> (*written when baby was four days old*)

If the woman is not married, the baby's father has sometimes come into the hospital with her. A friend or relative may come instead to offer emotional support and personal relationship for the birth.

Choosing an Obstetrician

Parents often ask help from a community childbirth education association or from hospital maternity supervisors on how to find an obstetrician and a pediatrician whose qualifications include interest in the new childbirth. Many doctors have adopted what they believe is a neutral attitude yet have not obtained the knowledge of how to be supportive. Frequently they are surprised if parents wish more than to be merely left alone to "do their thing." Others will offer information and help to parents.

If parents wish to know the interest of an obstetrician in prepared childbirth they can ask him how he feels about family-centered maternity care, prepared childbirth, or the Lamaze method of prepared childbirth. If he does not seem supportive or says that these questions can be answered later in the pregnancy, the chances are that he is not interested in being involved in an awake and participating childbirth with both parents present. If he says that he will take care of everything and not to worry, the woman cannot expect that he will understand her desires and help her achieve her goals.

Questions expectant parents sometimes ask which are *not* helpful are whether or not the woman can have natural childbirth and whether or not she can breast-feed. Answers to these questions tell the prospective patient little. The answers depend largely on the knowledge and preparation of the patient and doctor and the amount of support available in the hospital as well as possible medical factors. There are too many unknowns if the questions are presented in this way.

The attitude of the obstetrician is the important thing for parents. Will he offer his patient some support during labor if she should need it? How does he feel about leaving orders for medication to be given at the woman's request? How does he feel about routine spinals for prepared women? If the obstetrician seems supportive of education for childbirth other questions might be asked depending on the interest of the woman and her husband. How does he feel about husbands staying with their wives? Does he refer patients to childbirth education classes? How does he feel about breast feeding? Does he find that prepared childbirth and breast feeding work out well for most women? How often can the woman have her baby brought to her while in the hospital?

During the first visit to the obstetrician's office during pregnancy the husband should accompany his wife, if possible, to talk with the doctor. The doctor can then see not only the patient but the couple as expectant parents. The husband can ask any questions his wife may not have a chance to ask because she forgets or feels that she shouldn't ask for any more time. As the patient, she may feel a little more vulnerable than her husband.

Usually it takes very little time to ascertain an obstetrician's attitudes. If it is clear that his preference is to work with medicated, anesthetized patients in a conventional care system and that he will not help couples who wish the new kind of childbirth, the couples who desire a shared, participating experience will probably want to choose another obstetrician who understands their feelings and shares their goals.

II

Methods of Preparation: Breathing and Exercises

The techniques are really no big hassle. They are offered in detail here simply to show the range of workable techniques without the necessity of reading several books and then having to figure out for oneself the similarities and differences between Read, Lamaze, and other methods of preparation. As the techniques are compared, the reasons for using them become clearer. They then seem less like mumbo-jumbo with women doing this or that exercise, and breathing this way or that way with no apparent reason. Many of the techniques can be used for stress or pain not related to childbirth at all.

It is definitely unnecessary to know about all of the techniques described. Even teachers of childbirth education do not usually keep all of the techniques in their minds.

There are only certain things which are essential to know. Prepared childbirth requires that two people be in the labor room: the woman having the baby and someone to be with her, preferably her husband. The woman must be able to relax the muscles of her abdomen and the muscles of her vagina. She must lie in comfortable positions. During the dila-

tation stage of labor she must breathe in a controlled way to keep her diaphragm from interfering with the contracting uterus. During the delivery stage she must use her diaphragm actively to help push her baby out.

It was, I must admit, only by virtue of my wife's interest that she attended your class. I was almost dragged to the meeting that I attended. Because of her interest, though, I cooperated with her in her preparation for labor.

I was with her from the onset of labor . . . until about 4:00 A.M. the following morning, when she was about eight centimeters dilated and when she went up for an epidural. If I could have stayed with her for the delivery, we would have declined the anesthesia. She had no analgesic medication during the time I was with her.

In the course of my medical training through interneship I delivered perhaps seventy-five to one hundred babies. Even at the "Ivy League" center where I had this training we were very liberal with anesthesia. I have never seen a woman handle her labor with less agitation or less protest than my wife, despite all these medications. It was very clear that this graceful conduct of the labor came from her preparation through reading and through your classes. I must say that I was terribly impressed by what you have to offer women preparing for delivery, and that conviction had to break through a very strong wall of skepticism, I assure you. Perhaps most important is the tremendous emotional fulfillment the technique affords.

My wife is now doing fine and the baby is robust and

lovely. I thank you for what proved to be your con-
siderable helpfulness to us.

(*letter from young doctor-husband to childbirth
education instructor*)

What does labor feel like? What are the techniques used
and how do they work? Why do some classes teach different breathing than other classes? Couples facing childbirth
are facing much that is unfamiliar to them and they have
many questions.

The emphasis is on the "here and now" in every aspect of
the preparation. The class is geared to meet the present
needs of the couple, whatever doubts and fears may have
existed in the earlier lives of the men and women in classes.
Couples are given information, relief from anxiety, and
emotional support to promote confidence in themselves and
in each other as they prepared for birth and parenthood.

Emotional support and comfort measures are important
to the woman in labor but are not enough to keep her
comfortable in labor. Knowing about the physiology of birth
is important, too, but this is not enough by itself either.
The available methods of preparation for childbirth offer
physical conditioning exercises, relaxation techniques, and
breathing patterns which are reinforced by those who attend them in labor. The purpose of the techniques is simply
that of adding to the comfort of the woman in labor.

No one method of preparation has been shown to work
better than another. The techniques vary somewhat as they
are taught in different classes, but the theoretical interpretation of why they work is more variable than the general outline of what is actually taught. Sometimes methods

are combined if an instructor feels that the techniques of more than one method have something to offer. She may also describe the way in which a technique works in different ways. For example, effleurage (gentle, rhythmical stroking of the abdomen during a contraction), which originated with the Lamaze method, may be described by Read teachers primarily as a comfort measure to help relax the abdominal muscles. In a Lamaze class stressing psychoprophylaxis, the effleurage is described primarily as providing a focus of attention away from the contracting uterus, and as giving the woman something active to do which will not interfere with the necessary relaxation of the muscles near the uterus. This interpretation emphasizes distraction and activity rather than promoting comfort and relaxation.

The Contraction

The uterus contracts long before the woman goes into labor. It contracts even when she is not pregnant. During pregnancy she may be aware of Braxton Hicks contractions, which are often called practice contractions. They are felt as a tightening in the abdomen different from the sensations of the baby's movements. Although intense long-lasting contractions act to inhibit placental circulation, the mild and brief Braxton Hicks contractions are thought to aid the placental circulation as well as preparing the uterus for labor.

Masters and Johnson[1] found in their work that:

> Along with this series of contractions of the orgasmic platform, the uterus also contracts rhymically. Each

contraction [of the orgasm] begins at the upper end of the uterus and moves like a wave through the mid-zone and down to the lower or cervical end. Labor contractions prior to childbirth move similarly down-ward along the uterus in a wave-like progression, but are much stronger.

The mechanism which starts labor at a certain time is not entirely known, although labor can be artificially induced by the obstetrician. The distension of the uterus and the beginning dilatation of the cervix aided by the Braxton Hicks contractions lead to increased production of oxytocin. The oxytocin then encourages the contraction of the uterus.

During labor contractions the uterus, a hollow muscular organ, undergoes certain changes. As it tips forward against the abdominal wall, the upper portion of the uterus contracts most strongly. The lower portion is more passive. The longitudinal muscle fibers shorten during the contraction and remain shorter in length after the contraction has ceased, therefore tending to decrease the size of the uterine cavity, but there is also a compensatory relaxation and lengthening of circular muscle fibers around the mouth of the uterus in the lower segment. If there is an imbalance in the innervation (stimulation) of the uterus such as that which can be caused by fear and emotional stress, there could then be spasm of the circular fibers of the lower uterine segment instead of the normal relaxation. If the longitudinal muscle fibers must overcome unusual resistance of the lower, circular muscle fibers due to spasm, pain can be expected to be intensified. If the uterus contracts as it should, the baby's head moves deeper into the pelvis and the longitudinal fibers tend to draw the mouth of the uterus, the cervix, up over the baby's head.

After the cervix is dilated to the width of five fingers,

about four inches, the baby's head enters the birth canal. During the next stage of labor, the second stage, the contractions, aided by force from the abdominal muscles, begin to move the baby down the birth canal.

During the labor and delivery process the baby is completely passive. During the first stage of labor, while the cervix is dilating, the baby goes nowhere. He remains in the uterus just as he has for nine months.

During the second stage of labor the woman's body moves him down the birth canal. His head is turned as it meets bony obstacles. The wider part of the upper part of the pelvis is from side to side. The wider part of the lower part of the pelvis is from front to back, or anterior-posterior. At first the baby's head and body face to the side. As the contractions continue, his head is usually turned to face his mother's back. At this time his chin is tucked down on his chest. As he descends, the perineum around the outlet of the birth canal bulges and the mother often feels rectal pressure as the baby's head presses against the rectum. For a short time during this stage a splitting or burning sensation is often described. It is temporary and is compared by Hazell[2] to the feeling one gets when the dentist stretches one's mouth.

After the delivery of the head, which arrives face down, the baby turns his head to the side to line it up with the rest of his body, which is still unborn and which faces to the side. The shoulders emerge one at a time and the baby's body delivers immediately.

The contractions of the uterus during labor occur in a rhythmic fashion. They rise to a peak about halfway through the wave of the contraction. Occasionally they may peak two thirds of the way through the contraction. At first they last less than a minute. During most of the labor they last just about a minute. Women are usually relieved to learn that the interval of time between contractions is almost always longer than the duration of the contraction, except perhaps during transition at the end of the first stage. The untrained woman often thinks that the initial contractions she feels at the beginning of labor will get worse and worse, longer and longer. They do increase in rate and intensity, but the duration of the contractions remains about the same.

Women are taught to welcome the contractions as promoting progress toward birth instead of being afraid and making their muscles rigid. Weak contractions are less effective in dilating the cervix and may require hormonal stimulation to speed labor.

The length of the first stage of labor, the longest part, is unpredictable even though the length of each contraction is predictable. There is also no way of knowing the exact moment of onset of labor when the cervix begins to dilate, making accurate measurement of the length of the first stage difficult. The same woman having different babies may find the length of the first stage widely variable.

Transition at the end of the first stage has been described as lasting a half hour or fifteen contractions for a first baby. Some describe it as lasting a maximum of an hour or twenty contractions for a first baby. The time is less for second and subsequent babies. These contractions could even last as long as two minutes with only a minute of rest between each one for a short period of time.

During the second stage of labor leading to birth the contractions may last less than a minute with a couple of minutes between contractions. The second stage lasts from a few minutes to over an hour.

Grantly Dick-Read of England and Velvovski of Russia

felt that uterine contractions were not inherently painful but that pain was culturally induced through negative conditioning. Chertok[3] says that whether or not they are inherently painful does not matter. Besides, he says, there's no such thing as physiologic childbirth free from any cultural influence. He cites the advantages of preparation for childbirth as being the promotion of mental health and the suppression of pain. When discussing pain Vellay[4] makes an interesting comparison using the example of the biceps muscle. He says that if the muscle is contracted slowly pain will not result, but that if it is jerked it loses its physiological characteristics and it hurts.

Most women do experience labor contractions as painful, but with preparation they do not feel anything which could be called suffering under ordinary circumstances. Pain is a subjective sensation, but some women do actually describe painless labors, even if the labors are not devoid of sensation. Those describing psychoprophylactic preparation have even published figures as high as a third.

A pamphlet on pain from the Department of Health, Education and Welfare[5] says that muscles do not have the pain sensory organs of the skin, but muscles can cause severe pain when the products of muscular activity are not removed fast enough because of circulatory difficulty. The example of angina pectoris is given where lack of oxygen to the heart muscle causes great pain. Childbirth educators have always stressed the importance of adequate oxygen to the uterus through methods of breathing, although adequate oxygenation is not the sole reason for the breathing which is used. This pamphlet also says that in the stress of excitement, such as at a football game, a person can be injured without perceiving pain at the time because the excitement interferes with the perception of pain. This observation relates to the Lamaze method of preparation for childbirth in which the techniques taught are seen as inhibiting the perception of pain.

Methods of Preparation

Childbirth education classes may combine methods at times, and new techniques will continue to be tried by instructors and their students, by obstetricians and their patients. There are, however, several distinct approaches or methods. These tend to fall into two major divisions, the Read approaches and psychoprophylactic (or Lamaze) preparation. Both Read and Lamaze made fundamental contributions to childbirth education.

Read Preparation

This approach is not properly described as a method because the preparation was not fully developed as a system or method. As additions or changes are made in classes which are based on the teaching and philosophy of the late Dr. Grantly Dick-Read, the classes may be described as teaching a modified Read approach. If much of the knowledge from Lamaze training is included in the teaching it will probably be called a Lamaze class.

The Read approach is based on earlier work than the Lamaze method. It did not spread rapidly and was later eclipsed by the Lamaze method. Although the Read approach worked well for many, there were others who felt that it was too vague and that it also appeared to give the obstetrician an inadequate role, even making him feel not needed. Of course, the method did not remove the need for medical care, but this impression was created as a result of the then new and unfamiliar emphasis on the importance of the patient's role in medical care.

The Read approach is based on interrupting the fear-tension-pain cycle. Fear is described as leading to tension which then causes pain. Pain then leads to more fear. Read reduced fear by providing information and education. Muscular tension was reduced by lessening fear and by teaching bodily relaxation. Read discovered the fear-tension-pain cycle, as Chertok says, by "fruitful intuition." Chertok feels that the relationship between pain and tension requires physiological study, but Read did discover that childbirth was not necessarily painful, and that fear and anxiety are important factors in the pain of childbirth.

Read preparation includes the following:

1. Education about birth is emphasized. The teaching does not include the psychological analgesia of the Lamaze method which has taught a conditioned response to uterine stimuli. Read preparation, however, does offer deconditioning from earlier fears, myths, and misconceptions in the same way as does the Lamaze method.

2. The education about birth is discussed in the physiological language of voluntary muscle relaxation and physical conditioning exercises. The breathing techniques are soothing, aid bodily relaxation and the processes of birth. The preparation is based on working with body forces and feelings, and trusting the body to tell the woman who has been educated for childbirth how to respond. Read is known for his emphasis on relaxation and has been criticized for encouraging too much passivity, yet it is true that

many women have gone through labor comfortably with a kind of passive relaxation and without the use of any other technique.

3. Although the use of monitrices or labor coaches is less prevalent than in the Lamaze method, emotional support is very important and is offered by the husband, nurses, and doctor during the pregnancy, labor, and delivery.

4. Read-based classes have been characterized by more passivity of the woman than the classes teaching psychoprophylaxis. The woman turns inward toward what is happening inside her rather than looking for ways of distraction from uterine stimuli. Her eyes may be closed and she may drowse in a sleepy fashion. At present Read-based classes seem to emphasize more mental alertness, as taught in the Lamaze method, to enable the woman to meet each contraction as it comes, using the breathing and relaxation which she has been taught, but with more active control of her responses.

5. As in psychoprophylaxis, the breathing which is taught becomes more shallow and rapid as the contractions increase in intensity with panting breathing being used to prevent pushing prematurely at the start of the second stage of labor and during the delivery.

The Lamaze Method

The Lamaze method is the psychoprophylactic method first described in Russia which was brought to western Europe by Dr. Lamaze and adapted to his practice. It, too, has undergone some modification but remains fundamentally unchanged.

The word "psychoprophylaxis" is literally translated as "mind prevention." More liberally translated, it means prevention of pain.

As the method spread through the United States in the sixties, it added new thinking on prepared childbirth and gave a new vitality to education for childbirth. The Lamaze method seemed to have a greater mass applicability than Read teaching. Its added dimension was important to those who felt that they needed something more specific for comfort during labor than what had previously been offered.

Like the Read approach, Lamaze preparation includes the following:

1. It provides education about birth which includes teaching the importance of releasing uninvolved muscles.

2. It offers emotional support during labor and delivery. Lamaze teachers developed the role of the husband to provide specific coaching of Lamaze techniques during labor and delivery. The monitrice's role as labor coach became that of teaching the husband how to help his wife.

Lamaze preparation also offers other aspects.

1. An active, directive psychological analgesia is offered which is aimed at preventing pain as well as modifying the perception of pain. It is often said that psychoprophylaxis gives the woman something to do besides tense her muscles, whereas, with the untrained woman, whenever her uterus contracts a signal goes to her brain which then perceives the signal as pain. The perception of pain then gives the signal for fear and flight, an escape response causing generalized muscular tension. For the Lamaze-trained woman excitation (or stimulation) of the cortex of the brain has been thought to inhibit pain perception in the way that a physical ailment or injury is less noticeable during an engrossing

sporting event. This is another way of saying that if a meaningful stimulus is presented there is then an inhibition of transmission from other sensory modalities. The so-called cortical excitation for the Lamaze-trained woman is provided by controlled breathing. The breathing is accelerated during strong contractions to provide additional cortical excitation by using a higher level of conscious activity. The term "cortical excitation" is used less often now because there is no real knowledge of what actually occurs.

2. Besides this cortical excitation, as it was originally described, Lamaze instructors have felt that conditioned response was involved, although this term, too, is beginning to drop out of the language of childbirth education. Conditioned responses were discovered in Russia by Pavlov, who found that dogs could be trained to salivate at the sound of a bell. This discovery became incorporated into theories of learning. Lamaze teachers have taught that women in labor are conditioned to respond to the pressure of each contraction by doing controlled breathing and by letting go (dissociation) of uninvolved muscles. This *is* their response, but the words "automatic response" are beginning to be used instead of "conditioned response." Another learned or automatic response is that of panting to inhibit ill-timed pushing responses during transition and during the delivery of the baby's head.

During pregnancy the necessary responses are learned and practiced, not by the pressure of the contracting uterus, of course, but by the husband putting pressure on the inner thigh muscle of his wife's leg or by using some similar way of providing a stimulus.

3. Lamaze teaching includes the recognition of a physiological basis (like Read) for the techniques taught despite

the emphasis which has been placed on cortical excitation and conditioned response to prevent or relieve the pain of strong contractions. The method teaches that the pain of strong contractions may be caused by lack of oxygen to the hard-working uterine muscle. Spasm of uterine muscle fibers can even occur from inadequate oxygenation. It is felt, therefore, that controlled breathing can affect the quality of the uterine contraction itself. Muscular relaxation helps to conserve oxygen and to prevent fatigue.

4. The dynamics of the connection between relaxation and pain are complex just as the connections between breathing, emotions, and pain are complex. The Lamaze method recognizes the importance of the ability to release muscular tension just as the Read approach does. Discussion continues, however, about the form mental relaxation should take. Teachers of psychoprophylaxis feel that the passive concentration of Read may cause lowering of the level of awareness whereas the psychoprophylaxis of Lamaze raises the level of awareness, the focus of attention being on the breathing. Chertok says that a suggestive element is present in both approaches, but in neither is there hypnosis. Interestingly, though, it is not known whether hypnosis involves an unusually vigilant state of attention or a lessened degree of vigilance.

5. The method includes the use of some physical conditioning exercises, although fewer usually than classes not based on psychoprophylaxis. Exercises which are done are described in terms of stretching, strengthening, limbering, and aiding the release of uninvolved muscles. They are similar to those used in Read classes. Whether the teaching is Read or Lamaze, the relaxation, exercises, and breathing techniques all work to support each other in helping the woman gain control over her body.

6. Although psychoprophylaxis is a tool to be used to promote comfort, the Lamaze method is now described more in terms of interpersonal relationships and not only in terms of Pavlovian neurophysiology. There is also more discussion of the importance of the family. Bing describes her teaching of the husband to help his wife in labor as encouraging husband-wife communication and, more than that, the art of loving.

Lamaze teaching has been described by Vellay, Chabon, Chertok, Karmel, and Bing. The method taught by Lamaze teachers is basically the same, but there has been modification of the activity of the breathing, making it less deep and rapid so that there is less "huffing and puffing."

The Erna Wright Method

Erna Wright of England felt, although the Read approach had worked well for her personally, that many women needed something more specific. She went to France with Dr. Elliot Philipp to spend some time with Dr. Pierre Vellay to learn the Lamaze method. Later, back in England, working with Dr. Philipp, and associated with the National Childbirth Trust, she developed in her teaching a method based on psychoprophylaxis, but using less active breathing than was taught in the Lamaze method. She taught women to do no panting except when the woman was told by her doctor not to do any pushing. She divided the breathing techniques into four levels and taught women to "shift gears" as they moved from one level to another. As she promoted this method through her travels and her book,[6] it became known as the Erna Wright method. The breathing and exercises will be described in following pages.

The Psychosexual Method of Sheila Kitzinger

Sheila Kitzinger's teaching[7] is not based on psychoprophylaxis. In her association with the National Childbirth Trust in England she has developed a method of preparation for her classes based on using sensory memory as an aid in understanding and working with the body in preparation for birth. She arrived at her method from a sociological background, utilizing her experience in several cultures. She also used the Stanislavsky method of acting as a basis for her teaching of relaxation.

Her teaching is called the psychosexual method because she saw sexuality not only as genital but as part of a larger whole, including family relationships, birth, cuddling, feeding. She saw the importance of human relationships to the woman during her pregnancy. She recognized pregnancy as a vulnerable time, but also a fluid one in which the woman is capable of emotional growth. Women's feelings about themselves and their bodies, their families, their babies are interrelated and she adapted her teaching to offer couples specific help.

Marriage counseling in private interviews with couples became part of her teaching. At this time she showed the husband how to support his wife during childbirth and helped the wife learn to relax parts of her body toward his hand, to accept his support. The support was tactile as well as verbal. More than lip service was given to the importance of the language of touch.

Kitzinger also added to her classes specialized knowledge of the female pelvic floor and taught women how to gain better control over the openings in the pelvic floor and the muscle tissue up inside the vagina for more sensitive control of the descent and delivery of the baby.

Relaxation

Relaxation is usually the first technique taught in a child-birth class. It may seem strange that relaxation has to be taught, but it is not simple to do. The woman cannot ordinarily simply tell herself to relax whether she is in class or in the hospital during labor. The command to relax seems to invite tension. Relaxation is a conscious, active process requiring effort to maintain. It must not be confused with passivity.

Why does the woman in labor have to relax all her muscles when only certain muscles are involved in birth? One reason is that tension in one muscle tends to spread to other muscles. She will find, too, that tension disturbs her feeling of being in control of herself. She will, however, learn in class to tense certain muscles while relaxing others as, during labor, the uterine muscle will be contracting while other muscles are relaxed.

Jacobsen,[8] as a physiologist, says that muscular relaxation is a mechanical way of relieving pain. The progressive relaxation described by Jacobsen is taught in many classes based on Read teaching. Voluntary muscle groups are released one at a time. The woman may "talk" to her muscles as she lets go of muscles in her forehead, cheeks, eyes, jaws, neck, shoulders, upper arm, lower arm, wrist, fingers, other arm in the same way, abdomen, hips, thigh, calf, and toes.

Women may be told to focus on a pleasant "mind picture" or visual image of relaxed muscles while thinking of such words as "loose," "melt," or "heavy."

The degree of relaxation can be tested by the husband or instructor in class and, later, during labor, by the husband or nurse. They do this by picking up a wrist or ankle to see if it is limp, or they move a shoulder to test for tightness. In her classes Bing has the husband stand over his wife as she lies on the floor. One foot is on each side of her body. He grasps his wife's hands and lifts her elbows a couple of inches off the floor and swings the arms slowly as his wife releases all the muscles in her arms and shoulder. Tightness in the legs is tested by having the husband lift a knee off the pillow on which it is resting as his wife releases all of the muscles in the leg. She may then be told to release one or two limbs while contracting the muscles in the other limbs in a neuromuscular control exercise.

The physical contact of having an arm or leg tested helps the woman to become aware of tension. It may also offer a kind of physical reassurance which encourages relaxation, especially if she is told that she is relaxing well.

Relaxation is practiced in all of the comfortable positions listed in the section on comfort measures. If the woman is on her back her head will be on a pillow, her back rounded. The knees are bent, resting on pillows and rolled outward. Many women, however, prefer to sit up during much of the labor.

Bing and Enkin are among those teachers of childbirth who stress that it is important to use the words "contract" and "release" to replace the words "tense" and "relax." The word "contract" can be associated with the contractions of the uterus which are occurring during labor. Also the words "contract" and "release" are more immediate and specific than the words "tense" and "relax."

Kitzinger teaches relaxation by having women relax a little more with each exhalation breath. She has women "relax down their backs" and even gives them the mental image of "breathing down their backs" as the abdomen is allowed to spread to the sides. She uses such sensory images as, for example, visualizing a dress opening in back and slipping off both ends of a hangar to help attain relaxation of the shoulders, which are often hard to relax.

Exercise by itself does not promote relaxation, but relaxation can be learned by first tensing a muscle, then letting it go to the maximum extent possible. Consciously tensing a muscle and releasing it increases awareness of the degree of tension. If it is hard to release a muscle it helps to tighten it first. The muscle can then be released more completely. The woman may take a deep breath, inhaling as the muscle is tensed, and exhaling with a sighing breath as she lets it go. Exercises based on tensing and releasing muscles are done in all methods of preparation for childbirth.

Exercises

Many of the techniques described are listed under the heading of exercises. These may include relaxation techniques, neuromuscular control exercises to promote relaxation, physical conditioning exercises, and breathing techniques. There is an interrelationship among the techniques. For example, the breathing is often done in conjunction with neuromuscular control exercises, and the neuromuscular control exercises sometimes serve also the purpose of physical conditioning. The techniques all support each other, but for the purpose of clarity the techniques are listed under the headings of neuromuscular control exercises, physical conditioning exercises, comfort measures, and breathing methods. The following is not intended to be a list of all possible exercises, nor would one woman do all

of the exercises in each group. Instructors make selections
from each group when teaching couples in class. Each
technique used is practiced in class and at home.

Neuromuscular control Exercises

Although these exercises are associated with psychoprophylaxis, most writers and instructors describe some exercise of this type. Exercises may be called neuromuscular
control exercises, concentration exercises, or a dissociation
drill. During neuromuscular control exercises women learn
to tense certain muscle groups on command while releasing other groups.

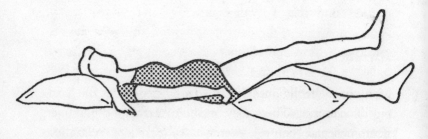

Bing, teaching the Lamaze method, has her students as
they lie on the floor respond to the command of "contract"
by tensing the right arm (shoulder, elbow, and fist) and
raising it before them a few inches from the floor. The
arm is tightened as much as possible and held until the command is given to release it. The arm then goes limp and
drops to the floor. This exercise is done with each of the
arms and legs. It is then done with both arms, then with
the arm and leg on the same side, and, finally, with the arm
and leg on opposite sides. It is called a concentration-relaxa-
tion exercise.

Wright describes an active decontraction drill in which the woman breathes in as she tenses a muscle, then blows out as she relaxes or decontracts it. This exercise is done with arm, leg, mucles around vagina, upper chest, shoulder muscles, and face.

She follows this exercise by teaching an active dissociation drill in which the left arm is contracted for forty-five seconds using the deepest level of breathing. The same procedure is followed with the right arm, then with right arm and right leg, left arm and left leg, and finally asymmetrically, using the arm and leg on opposite sides of the body. This drill is combined with breathing: three breaths in level A, four to six breaths in level B, eight to ten breaths in level C, then down through C, B, and A again while making sure that no other muscles have joined in the contraction except the designated ones. It is called the dissociation drill in opposition to the condition of muscle association in which the contraction of the uterus causes generalized bodily tension.

Miller, not teaching psychoprophylaxis, teaches his patients concentration exercises which follow the above pattern of arm, leg, and then symmetric and asymmetric tensing of arms and legs. He recommends holding the contraction for twenty seconds, and stresses as do other teachers that the heels must be pointed down when tensing the legs to avoid cramps in the calf of the leg.

Kitzinger, who does not teach psychoprophylaxis either, uses differential relaxation. She contracts, then releases abdominal muscles, calf muscles, and other muscles. She then tenses an arm, raising it slightly from the floor with the fist clenched, followed by release. This is done with the leg on the same side, then the leg on the opposite side. She does not, however, raise legs from the floor as Wright does because she feels that this places too much pull on the abdominal muscles and lower spine.

Earlier, Goodrich and Heardman had also described this exercise, although Heardman did not describe the asymmetric tensing and releasing.

The Maternity Center Association* booklet available to parents called "Preparation for Childbearing" advocates using conscious relaxation in which the woman systematically tightens and loosens groups of muscles beginning with the toes and working up to the face in a progressive relaxation exercise during which parts of the body are released one at a time.

As can be seen, there is more than one way of obtaining the benefits of this type of exercise.

Physical Conditioning Exercises

The physical conditioning exercises have the purposes of stretching, strengthening, and limbering, and are designed to increase comfort during pregnancy as well as during childbirth. They fall into one of four groups: (1) stretching, relaxing, and strengthening inner thigh muscles and limbering pelvic joints; (2) strengthening back and abdominal muscles to relieve backache and to help in carrying baby in correct position in the pelvis; (3) gaining control over and strengthening pelvic floor muscles; and (4) body mechanics and other exercises which may be done to promote comfort during pregnancy. All classes will have one

* Located at 48 East 92nd Street, New York, N.Y. 10028.

or more exercises from each of the first three groups. The exercises are simple to do and the muscle stretch feels good.

1. *Tailor sitting* has always been associated with natural childbirth classes. The woman sits on a hard surface cross-legged with her back straight but slightly rounded to avoid back strain. Often the husband is taught to place his hands on the outside of his wife's thighs. She then tries to open

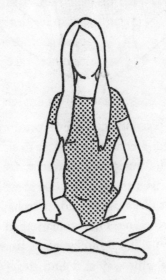

them against the resistance he provides. Vellay has the woman separate her knees, bring them together, and then separate them again.

If the soles are placed together and drawn toward the body more stretch is provided. The pelvic floor can be relaxed and even bulged at the same time as the woman gets the feeling of allowing space for the baby to pass through.

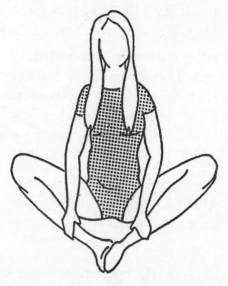

At first these positions may be uncomfortable, but with practice they offer a comfortable way to sit. After practice the stretch on the inner thigh muscles feels good.

Bing also describes another exercise in which the woman sits on the floor, legs apart and stretched forward, and knees turned outward. The woman then leans forward between her legs. This exercise also stretches the lower back in much the same way as does the exercise which used to be taught in which the woman lies on her back and raises her head while drawing her knees up toward her shoulders.

The tailor sitting exercise with the soles together can also be done while lying on the back. The knees are drawn up and flopped outward as the soles are drawn up to the pubis.

Classes teaching psychoprophylaxis do another exercise which stretches the inner thigh muscles. Bing has her students lie on their backs with pillows under the head and knees and arms at the sides. After taking a breath one leg is raised slowly as high as is comfortable. A breath is taken

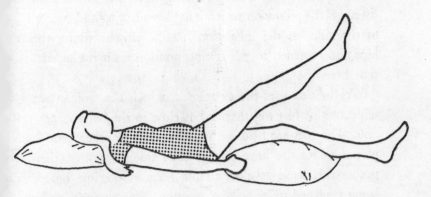

in through the nose. The leg is then lowered slowly while exhaling through the mouth. Following this exercise the arms are extended to the sides at right angles. The leg is raised, keeping the knee straight, as the breath is inhaled, and lowered gently outward as close to the hand on the same side as is possible during the exhalation breath. The leg is then raised again and lowered to its original position while breathing as before.

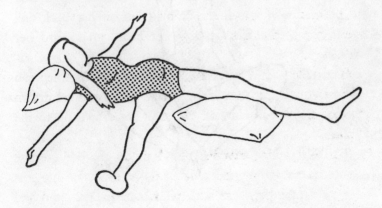

Classes using the Wright manual do a similar exercise. One leg is lifted with a straight knee while breathing in and dropped again while breathing out. The leg is then lifted off the pillow on which it has been resting and swung to the side on the inhalation breath without tilting the hips and returned to the resting position with the exhalation breath.

Wright also uses the exercise in which the woman sits with soles of feet together and as close to the body as possible. The feet are held with one hand. The other hand is placed under the knee on the same side. The knee then pushes this hand as close to the floor as possible before being returned to its original position. This exercise is also done using both knees at once.

2. The *squatting position* is another exercise to provide stretch. It is used less often now but was originally as-

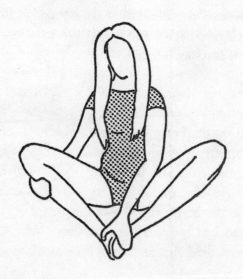

sociated with the Read approach to childbirth. The practice of the semi-squatting position which is rehearsed for the delivery serves the same purpose. Some women find this exercise very difficult to do. It is done by placing the feet about eighteen inches apart with toes pointed slightly outward, bending the knees with the back straight, and going down to the floor as low as possible while keeping the feet flat on the floor as toddlers do. At first it is necessary to hang onto a doorknob or the husband's hand for balance, but this exercise becomes easier to do with practice. It gives a great deal of stretch and, as pregnancy advances, the woman feels that the baby is very low in the pelvis and close to the outside world.

Kitzinger advises against remaining in this position for long because of possible interference with the circulation in the legs. She recommends bouncing on the heels instead.

3. The *pelvic rock exercise*, in some form, is used in all classes, and among its benefits is that of supporting the baby adequately in the pelvis during pregnancy. It is also used after delivery to tighten the abdominal muscles. It can be done lying on the back, standing, kneeling on hands and knees, or while lying in a side position.

In the standing position the exercise is done by placing one hand on the lower back and the other hand over the baby. First the abdominal muscles are tightened and the buttocks tucked under while the shoulders remain level and the knees are relaxed, The abdominal muscles and the muscles in the buttocks are then released. In this way the pelvis is rocked backward and forward. When not doing the exercise the buttocks should be tucked under and the abdominal muscles drawn in so that the baby does not rest on a sagging abdomen.

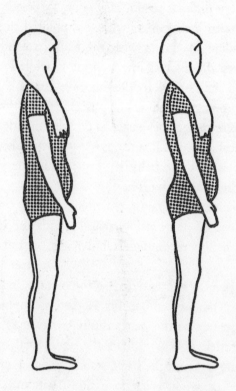

The pelvic rock is done on all fours by making a square box with the hands parallel and the shoulders over the hands. The buttocks are pulled under, then released, but the back should not be allowed to really cave in as the pelvis is rocked.

When the pelvic rock is done on the back as in most Lamaze classes the knees are bent so that the feet are firmly

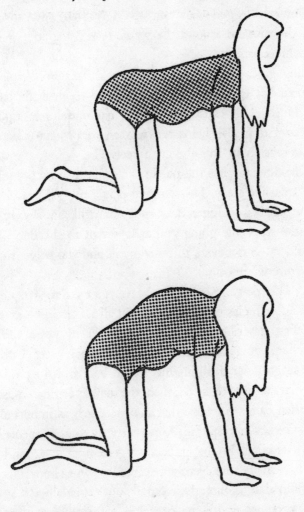

on the ground. The back is pressed against the floor, pulling in the abdomen at the same time and letting the buttocks lift slowly off the floor. Muscles are then released, allowing the small of the back to come off the floor.

The stiff-legged walk tilts the pelvis sideways to exercise the muscles around the waist. It is a variation taught in some classes.

Bing gives an additional abdominal exercise. After the woman has exhaled she blows out the residual air left in the lungs. This causes the abdominal muscles to tighten. Of course, it also helps the woman to become aware of what tension in the abdomen feels like.

Kitzinger teaches the pelvic rock on all fours as arching the back like a cat. The standing pelvic rock she teaches as belly dancing which is done, not as a drill, but slowly and luxuriously while going gradually down to the floor. The shoulders do not have to remain still and the pelvis rotates in a circular motion.

4. The *pelvic floor exercise* is referred to frequently in childbirth classes and is taught in all classes. The exercise was first described by Kegel a number of years ago for treatment of female urinary incontinence. Kegel found that surgery for this difficulty could be avoided by the use of this exercise to strengthen the pelvic-vaginal muscles. He then came to realize that the exercise was important to feminine sexual response. Apparently there were specialized nerve endings in the pubococcygeus muscle around the vagina. Finally, the exercise became known as important for childbirth. It is directly related to the birth itself as this muscle comes under the conscious control of the woman having a baby.

Its purposes in a childbirth class include that of reducing feelings of discomfort and congestion during pregnancy when the weight of the baby may tend to interfere with circulation, especially if the woman stands or sits for a period of time. This congestion is also associated with the possibility of hemorrhoids. The pelvic floor exercise tends to aid circulation in the pelvic floor as well as acting to tighten the pelvic floor to support the pelvic organs before and after birth. Of course, overstretched tissues can be repaired surgically later on, but it is important to avoid the need for this. Besides maintaining muscle tone, the exercise promotes elasticity and the ability to release the muscles in the pelvic floor during birth. This release is not only at the surface but also is deep inside. The ability to release these muscles decreases the amount of resistance offered to the baby's head. As the woman attains conscious control over these muscles the delivery is eased for mother and baby.

The pelvic floor is the area between the thighs and between the vagina and rectum. Some of the muscle fibers in this area pass around the rectum and also around the vagina and urethra in a figure-eight pattern. Although there is a muscular connection between the openings in the pelvic floor, it is nevertheless possible to differentiate between the contraction of the rectum and the contraction of the vagina. If the muscles of either opening are contracted slowly enough, it is possible to contract the muscles around one of the openings with little motion of the other.

Kitzinger has done the most work in adapting the exercise for childbirth. She describes several exercises which can be done. She has her students learn to contract and relax the muscles around the vagina with the inner thigh muscles contracted and then with them relaxed, then with the gluteal muscles in the buttocks contracted and next with them relaxed. The untrained woman in childbirth may tense the buttocks as she feels the sensations of the baby's head coming down. The tension can then spread to the perineum and it usually does.

The ability to contract at will the muscles in the perineum can be tested by stopping urination in mid-stream, but this is only a check. Keeping the distinction between elimination and birth is important.

Kitzinger also describes the tensing of vaginal muscles as like an elevator going up. The muscles are gradually drawn in more and more as deep inside as possible, then equally slowly released all the way down and then bulged at the "basement floor." The muscles are then tightened again slightly to a state of normal tone just as the mouth is not left hanging open in a totally relaxed state.

5. *Body mechanics and other exercises* may be given in addition to those which stretch the thigh muscles, rock the pelvis, and exercise the pelvic floor. They are more likely to be given in a class which has more than six sessions and which is not based on psychoprophylaxis. For example, the woman may be shown how to roll over on her side before getting out of bed or how to lift heavy objects with her back straight. For aching legs, or to prevent varicosities, she might be shown the right-anglo position with her legs up against a wall or a position which will raise the hips. For upper back discomfort a shoulder-circling exercise may be suggested, or for tired ankles a foot-circling exercise might be suggested.

Comfort Measures

Relaxation techniques are the basic comfort measures which are used in conjunction with the breathing techniques. Additional comfort measures are comfortable body positions, back rubs, and effleurage.

1. The woman in labor may choose one of the following body positions: (1) relaxing in a chair with head and forearms supported; (2) lying on her back with all limbs including her arms if possible supported by pillows and the

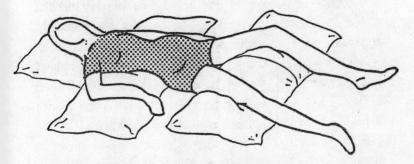

bed slightly raised; (3) sprawled sideways in a "running position" with the bed flat and the baby resting on the bed,

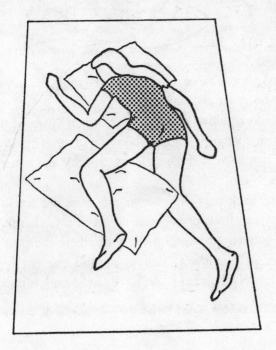

the lower arm down and in back, a pillow between the knees and one pulled under the head and chest; (4) up on all fours for back pain, perhaps doing the pelvic rock; (5) sitting straight up with pillows under separated knees in a cross-legged position and back supported; and (6) leaning

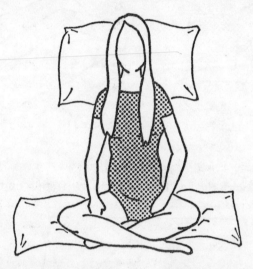

forward on a table or chair back, allowing the lower part of the body to go limp.

Instead of pillows a Hexham air bolster* may be used. It is a white, spongeable rubber bolster 32 inches by 16 inches which is inflated to three-quarters capacity and deflated for storage.

2. For back pain the woman can press her fist into the small of her back or she can be given a back rub, using strong counter pressure on the spot where the pain is felt whether in the lower back or around the tail bone. A clean tennis ball placed in the small of the back is now being

* National Childbirth Trust, Hexham, Northumberland, England.

used to give the needed pressure. The spot may move down as labor progresses. Sometimes an X marked with a ball-point pen is used to mark the spot. Pressure by itself can be used, or the heel of the hand can be moved in a slow, circular motion. Another way of giving a back rub is to move the hand slowly up and off the back. The motion must be slow and rhythmical. Powder is used to avoid skin irritation.

If, during transition, the pressure is felt at the rectum, Bing recommends taking a section of the sheet and pressing it against the rectum to support the tissues for immediate relief. This pressure might be felt as the baby's head starts to come down and move forward.

3. Effleurage is a light stroking of the abdomen done by the woman herself or by someone who is with her during labor. Wright uses the tips of the fingers, moving the fingers of both hands up the midline of the abdomen, around the top of the baby, and down around the sides. Another method she suggests uses the fingers of one hand to circle the entire abdomen.

Bing and Chabon do the effleurage similarly. While doing the first level of breathing, the hands are moved up the abdomen on the inspiration breath and then down to the starting point during the exhalation breath.

Pressure can be used as needed on pelvic bones or aching legs, but the effleurage should be gentle and not done with a rubbing motion. Women are sensitive to pressure on the uterus during labor. Rubbing the abdomen may cause pain, the result being that more active breathing will be required to cope with the contraction. This in turn may cause hyperventilation.

Breathing Methods

Breathing is a physical act which can represent an emotional state. Gasping, irregular breathing is associated with panic and can promote fear and pain. Breathing, emotions, and body functioning are related.

Lowen, as a psychiatrist,[9] finds that emotional disturbance may cause immobilization of the diaphragm and tightened muscles, including tightened abdomen and shoulders and a narrowed chest. His therapy includes the teaching of deep, relaxed breathing.

Yoga teaching describes controlled breathing in conjunction with the attainment of a high degree of relaxation as muscles are tensed slowly in a single contraction and released during prolonged relaxation.

Many of the answers about the connections between breathing, pain, and emotions are not known. In childbirth classes the breathing methods which are given teach women to coordinate the breathing with muscular release and with the rhythm of the contraction. The breathing methods for use during labor and delivery are often called breathing exercises because they involve learning and respiratory muscle activity.

In the Lamaze method the controlled breathing is a conditioned response to uterine stimuli. It is also soothing if the woman can hear a slight sound as she breathes. Concentrating on the breathing helps to keep disturbing thoughts from coming into her mind at this time.

Breathing activity, which is so much under conscious control, controls the action of the diaphragm. The diaphragm extends horizontally across the body, dividing the chest and abdominal cavities. When it descends during an inspiration breath, it turns up somewhat at the outer edges like an umbrella held upside down. In deep breathing it descends lower into the abdominal cavity than it does in shallow breathing. It is not easy to become aware of the diaphragm, although sometimes it may be possible to feel it move downward during an inspiration breath if the fingers are placed at the arch where the ribs come together.

As labor progresses the uterus becomes more sensitive to pressure from the diaphragm as well as to any pressure exerted by the abdominal muscles. The uterus does need oxygen, however, and, unlike running or physical activity involving many muscles, the contraction of the uterine muscle may not stimulate adequate breathing.

Another aspect of the subject of breathing must be considered. Rapid, gasping inspiration breaths or the blowing out of too much air in panic result in an alteration in the oxygen-carbon dioxide balance in the body, thereby affecting the acid-base balance of the body. If too much carbon dioxide is lost, the alkalinity of the mother's blood is increased, resulting in a seemingly paradoxical lack of oxygen available to the baby. This situation also causes dizziness in the mother and tingling of the hands or feet. This hyperventilation can occur in situations which have nothing to do with having a baby. Frightened, anxious people sometimes hyperventilate and may even come to hospital emergency rooms, fearing that they are ill. Hyperventilation is corrected by holding the breath for a few moments or by rebreathing some carbon dioxide. This is done by breathing with the hands cupped over the nose and mouth. The awake, cooperating woman in labor is taught to breathe in a way that helps to avoid the possible hyperventilation which may occur with the untrained woman.

A childbirth class teaches approximately three or four breathing techniques to be done during contractions to cope with labor as it progresses. Observers in the labor room of the hospital often cannot tell whether the woman is using the psychoprophylaxis of Lamaze or another method.

First Breathing Technique Used in Labor

The deepest, most relaxed type of breathing is done in early labor. All of the lung space is filled with air as the breath is slowly and steadily inhaled and exhaled.

The major difference in the teaching of the first breathing method to be used in labor has been the discussion of whether the breath was to be an abdominal breath or a chest breath. The two kinds of breathing are identified in the following way. While lying on the back, one hand is placed on the chest, the other on the abdomen. During an abdominal breath the abdomen will rise as the breath is drawn in. During a chest breath the chest will rise. When told to do relaxing breathing, people have a tendency to prefer one over the other. Both abdominal and chest breathing work if the breathing is slow, deep, and controlled, and if the body is relaxed.

Abdominal breathing was originally associated with Read preparation but was never used in the Lamaze method, which teaches chest breathing. Some of the teachers who do not emphasize psychoprophylaxis use abdominal breathing and some use chest breathing. Some simply tell their students to take a complete breath. Kitzinger teaches chest breathing, but at the same time teaches the release of the abdomen. She suggests having the mental image of breathing through the vagina also.

Many teachers feel that chest breathing is preferable because, if the diaphragm is down and the abdomen bulged as in abdominal breathing, more pressure is placed on the uterus than if chest breathing is done and the lower part of the body left alone. Also, many find abdominal breathing difficult to do as labor progresses and the uterus is in a more forward position, although by then the woman has probably moved to a higher breathing level. And yet many have found abdominal breathing to be comfortable during labor and that it supports uterine activity without interfering with the contraction. They have even used it with comfort almost up to transition with no need to raise the breathing level at all. It may be that some women are natural abdominal breathers who relax well during this breathing. Possibly, too, they are taller, longer-waisted women.

When discussing abdominal breathing and its current lack of popularity, it is well to remember that the so-called Birth Bubble is based on the principle of lifting the abdomen off the uterus in the same way as does abdominal breathing. Some hospitals have these Birth Bubbles which fit over the patient's abdomen. The abdominal wall is lifted by suction. The purpose is to ease and speed labor without need for the usual amounts of drugs. It is used for women who have not had a childbirth course.

Abdominal breathing is taught as slow breathing, the rate being four to six or seven breaths per minute. It has even been taught as done with a single long, slow breath with the peak of the breath at the peak of the contraction. If needed, a "catch" breath is taken. The mental image may be one of the cervix opening.

Since both chest and abdominal breathing work, the important factors seem to be that the abdominal muscles are not contracted and the breathing is gentle, slow, deep, and comfortable. It is started when the woman needs something besides relaxation alone to keep her comfortable during the contractions. It is most likely to be done with the breath taken in through the nose and exhaled through the mouth. The reasons for specifying nose or mouth relate to the fact that breathing through the nose causes more resistance to air intake than when the mouth is used and breath is taken in more slowly. On the other hand, mouth breathing is faster when quick intake of breath is desired as later in labor when the breathing rate is increased. Mouth breathing has the advantage of providing a slight sound, but it is also drying to the mouth if used for long periods.

Bing and Chabon teach the Lamaze method by using six to nine breaths per minute in slow, deep chest breathing. The breath is inhaled through the nose and exhaled through the mouth as though blowing on a bowl of soup. Bing is now suggesting a whistle on the exhalation breath. The eyes are focused on some point outside of herself to help the woman keep in contact with reality. She has a mental image of the contraction as seen on a diagram which shows the rise and fall of the contraction. To this is added a light effleurage described in the section on comfort measures.

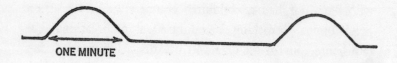

ONE MINUTE

This deep breathing is also used later in labor as a "cleansing breath" just before each contraction starts, and again a deep relaxing breath as the contraction finishes. The woman feels the need for these breaths, they help her relax, and they help define the beginning and ending of each contraction.

The first level of breathing is used as long as it feels comfortable. It is sometimes said to work up until two fingers (or 4 centimeters) dilatation, but no arbitrary time can be given for moving up to the next level of breathing. The ability to maintain relaxation is a factor in the length of time one can remain comfortable with quiet breathing. As the level of breathing changes, most women find it helpful to place their hands on the abdomen, ribs, or upper chest, according to which level they are using.

Second Breathing Level Used in Labor

When something more than the deep breathing of the first level is needed, the breathing is made shallower so that all of the lung capacity is no longer used. The rate must, therefore, increase. The increased rate and the changed level provide more activity and require more concentration on the breathing.

Some instructors teach the next level as one which uses the rib muscles and is a little higher than the chest breathing. Teaching based on Read or on the Erna Wright method describes this level as intercostal, sternal-costal, or costal-sternal. Costal means ribs. Sometimes it is called mid-chest breathing. It is called level B in the Erna Wright method. It is not used in the Lamaze method. Bing's first level may be done as deep chest breathing or visualized as a little higher, like rib breathing.

With each inhalation breath the ribs swing out. If the fingers are placed in the space between the ribs it is possible to feel the ribs swing out. The breath is exhaled through flabby lips blowing slightly. The rate depends on the need felt by the woman who is doing it.

Third Breathing Level Used in Labor

Instructors who do not use *both* deep chest breathing and rib breathing, or abdominal and rib breathing, go directly from the first breathing level, consisting, most likely, of a slow deep chest breathing, to an upper chest type of breathing.

As labor advances there is the wish to reduce further the motion of the diaphragm. For this level of breathing the rib cage does not move and the shoulders are kept down. If any urge to push is felt at this time (and it may not be), the breath is blown out to inhibit the urge to push. Sometimes women take a cushion of air and breathe on top of this cushion of air. The breathing is at the level of the breastbone or above it. High chest breathing is described in psychoprophylactic (Lamaze) teaching methods and in teaching not based on the Lamaze method. Miller tells his patients to take about 100 breaths per minute. The rate of breathing may be given as ranging between 60 and 150 breaths per minute. The panting breathing at this stage, earlier characteristic of Lamaze teaching, has been replaced by light and rapid breathing. This has been found workable and to reduce unnecessary fatigue. Fatigue makes the need for medication more likely and there is no need to induce fatigue unnecessarily. Vellay describes the breathing as being audible, but not panting.

The contraction changes in intensity during the course of each contraction. Therefore the breathing rate, and even the level, may be changed during a contraction to adapt to the changes in intensity. It may be accelerated as the contraction increases in intensity and decelerated as the contraction subsides.

There is always the deep, cleansing breath taken before and after each contraction which helps to define the beginning and end of each contraction and also aids muscle relaxation.

Kitzinger describes mouth-centered breathing which is above the level of the sternum and above the level of the throat, too, because the breath might catch in the throat. The breathing which she describes is felt in the mouth and is so gentle that she calls it hummingbird breathing. The jaw is dropped and the head is slightly forward.

The booklet prepared by the Maternity Center Association advocates what it calls modified complete breathing. A complete breath is taken. Each of the next four or five breaths is made a little shallower than the preceding breath. Then, as the contraction wanes, each of the next four or five breaths is made a little stronger and deeper. This type of breathing is not high and rapid.

Wright moves up the ladder of breathing levels during a single contraction. Level C is taught by having the woman place her hands on her breastbone so that the main effort will be felt there. She mouths the word "out" with each exhalation breath, concentrating on keeping the cheeks taut. During a contraction three breaths in level A are suggested, three to four in level B, then level C breathing for fifteen to twenty-five seconds, three to four breaths in level B again, and finally finishing with three level A breaths. If the contraction is strong the distraction techniques of level D can be used at the peak of the contraction.

Elisabeth Bing and Dr. Murry Enkin described the following breathing for advanced labor at a recent workshop. The breathing is done in the mouth, but the mouth is not open very wide to avoid drying the mouth. The breath is audible and whistled as it is exhaled. It is done in the 4/4 rhythm of "Yankee Doodle" or a similar tune, emphasizing slightly the first of each four breaths. The woman inhales and exhales on each beat of the tune. The rate is not as rapid as some methods describe. It can be rehearsed by holding the arm out in front stiffly for a minute while doing the breathing. As the contraction finishes the arm is released, a cleansing breath is taken, and the woman is told to smile. Smiling during a contraction is helpful in raising the breathing up into the chest. The time seems shorter if the husband tells her when the contraction is a quarter over, half over, and three quarters over in addition to telling her when the contraction starts and finishes.

Transition

The woman usually needs to be coached through each contraction. There is often an urge for some kind of activity after having worked so diligently to remain relaxed, and yet the activity must not interfere with the work of the uterus, which has still not entirely dilated the cervix. To indulge this desire for activity many women use distraction techniques at this time, including those who up to this point have preferred to relate their response more directly to the contraction itself.

The rhythm of a song may be tapped out on the thigh, the words of a song may be mouthed or even sung. Counting may be done with the breathing. Women may feel a bit foolish when they start to practice these techniques for distraction, but the techniques have been found to meet a need during transition.

In general, the rapid shallow breathing already described is used. Occasionally the breathing may be a little deeper in a rhythmical, shallow, panting kind of breathing. The second type of breathing used during transition is a shallow blowing. This is added because sometimes, though not always, the urge to push is beginning to be felt. This desire to push cannot be indulged because the dilatation is not yet complete. If the breath were to be inhaled deeply and held, the woman in transition might find herself pushing in spite of herself. The uterus continues to contract, but the woman avoids adding any bearing-down kind of pressure by doing panting or shallow blowing. The blowing must be shallow or a push will occur. The rapid blowing does not control the urge to push if the desire is strong, but it does inhibit the ability to push.

Whatever breathing method is chosen for transition must be practiced in the sitting and in the side positions because the woman in transition is likely to be sitting or she may be lying on her side.

A pant-blow type of breathing is often taught for transition. Bing feels that about six fast panting breaths through the mouth before the blow through pursed lips works out about right for most women. The Maternity Center booklet recommends the modified complete breathing previously described, but puffing gently every third or fourth breath. Vellay describes a breathing which is almost panting, interrupting this breathing to blow when the contraction demands it. He suggests counting or humming a tune as possible tools for distraction.

Some classes suggest using a one-two, one-two slump. The counting is done during the breathing followed by a slump when the rib cage is allowed to collapse. This technique can be seen to be similar to the pant-pant-blow technique.

Kitzinger continues the hummingbird breathing done in the mouth with the diaphragm raised and the abdomen relaxed. If the breathing gets tangled or any pushing urge is felt, the air is blown out and a new breath drawn in.

The woman can also lie on her side panting shallowly, her elbow on her upper hip and patting her abdomen. She blows when necessary.

Wright does level D breathing at the height of the contraction. The breathing is done lightly and rapidly, not concentrating on the breathing but just letting it happen. The woman concentrates on tapping out the rhythm of a tune while mouthing the words.

Common elements can be seen in the techniques just described. It would be impossible to say that one works better than another. They all work, but people who try them tend to have preferences. Whatever technique is to be used must be practiced. The major difference in techniques for transition revolves around how much activity or cortical stimulation is necessary. For example, some women do not tap the thigh as they count but prefer to slap it.

Two other techniques for transition have been used with success. One Lamaze group teaching classes describes a "ha-hooh" kind of breathing. The woman turns her head to the side as she whispers "ha" and back to the front as she says "hooh." This is done very actively and rapidly.

Another technique has been used in some back labors where the contraction is felt in the back. The woman lies on her side with her back curved. She does the pelvic rock. Breathing more slowly than many women find possible during transition, she breaths in as she pulls the middle of her back in and she breathes out as her back is again curved out.

The transition period is not an obstetrical entity. In obstetrics it is simply the end of the first stage of labor. Childbirth educators do describe it as a stage of labor for women having a conscious and cooperating birth experience because it feels different and because it requires specific techniques for coping with the feelings at that time. Yet there are women who never use these transition techniques at all and who wonder why there is so much emphasis on techniques for transition.

Second Stage of Labor and the Delivery

During this stage body position, breathing, muscular activity, and muscular relaxation are all involved. It is no longer necessary to keep the body entirely relaxed. The woman uses her muscles to help push her baby out into the world.

At this time she does one of two types of breathing during the contractions. In one type she takes deep breaths and then holds her breath. This is the only time during childbirth that the breath is held during a contraction because during the dilatation stage breath-holding would invite unwanted tension. During this second stage, however, as the baby is moved down the birth canal, the deep breath taken in and held lowers the diaphragm, allowing the mother to lean on it to help push her baby out. She exerts force from behind the baby's body.

The second type of breathing done during this stage is the panting already mentioned. Panting not only prevents the mother from pushing prematurely during transition but also keeps her from pushing during the delivery of the baby's head when the extra force from the voluntary muscles is not desired. She pushes to move the baby down but not during the delivery. When the obstetrician says, "Stop pushing," she translates the command into immediate panting. She breathes in and out quickly, this time dropping her head and shoulders back on the pillow and letting her arms fall back. Just as earlier during transition she must be helped, coached, and informed on the progress of dilatation, during the delivery she must also be coached. Without a mirror she cannot see the descent of the baby. She cannot know of it unless she is told. She does not know that the baby's head is on the perineum, that it is crowning. If she feels a smarting, stretching sensation she may ask whether she should pant, but not all women feel this sensation.

During the pushing stage the mother is propped up almost at a 45-degree angle. She should never be flat on her back. The semi-sitting position aids comfort and avoids possible pain. It is important also to the fetal circulation because the flat position tends to cause compression of a major maternal blood vessel due to the weight of the uterus. Thirdly, the semi-sitting position helps to prevent unnecessary difficulty in pushing, a difficulty which may result in the need for spinal anesthesia or even, rarely, an otherwise unnecessary Caesarean section. A pillow folded in half will give extra elevation if there is a shortage of pillows in the hospital. The husband or nurse can also place an arm under the woman's shoulders to hold her forward during a contraction. As the contraction begins to build she is raised up. She puts her arms around her knees with elbows out to the side to give room for the baby. She takes one or two deep, cleansing breaths and exhales them. She then takes a breath and holds it. As the contraction builds she pushes down and forward through a relaxed vagina. If she needs another breath she exhales the first one quickly and takes another. She may need two or three breaths during the contraction. The breath is held firmly and not allowed to escape with a groaning sound. This would not only dissipate the force of the push and place strain on the throat but would also make a groaning sound as though she were in pain.

The pushing stage is often mistakenly compared with the pushing done to empty the rectum. The description of pushing in such terms can cause incorrect pushing for childbirth, although the two types are related. Rectal pressure is commonly felt as the head comes down, but this is not always so. During the second stage of labor the push comes from in front on top of the abdomen. The mother pushes with the focal point on top of the uterus, directing the push downward as in a piston action. She pushes downward and forward toward the obstetrician. If she were lying flat on her back and expelling the baby as though emptying the rectum, the baby would be pushed over the rough spinal bones and against the rectum.

The second stage is taught fairly uniformly with no significant variations among the methods of preparation except for the method described by Kitzinger. There is one exception. While many teachers tell women to put the chin on the chest to prevent escape of air while pushing, Bing tells her students to simply put the head forward, feeling that placing the chin on the chest produces unnecessary redness of the face because of its effect on circulation.

The second-stage positioning and breathing methods are rehearsed during pregnancy, and the perineum is bulged, but most women in pregnancy do not actually practice anything more than very gentle pushing.

Kitzinger handles the pushing stage and delivery in the following way. She does not feel that the forceful pushing usually taught for the second stage is always necessary, especially with second or subsequent babies. She describes a gentler pushing activity as the baby is squeezed gently and easily down the birth canal. For second or subsequent babies she suggests that the mother might want to try a minimum push. A couple of deep breaths are taken, followed by mouth-centered breathing instead of holding the breath as in the maximum push. She asks her doctor whether she should push, perhaps do a minimum push, or blow the contraction away without pushing at all.

Kitzinger has made another change. She pushes with a relaxed abdomen instead of the contracted abdominal muscles usually advocated. She keeps the arms relaxed, too. The mouth is not closed as taught by most instructors. If the woman feels tense, she opens her mouth slightly. A relaxed, smiling mouth may help open up the lower part of the body.

She feels that if the arms are supported by pillows there is no need for tense arms to grip the legs during a contraction. If the abdominal muscles are contracted, she feels that the woman is more likely to find herself with a tight vagina. Readers might want to experiment for themselves by pretending to push a baby down through the pelvis with contracted muscles, then with released abdominal muscles. If the muscles are released during the pushing action, a hand placed on the lower abdomen will be pushed outward.

How Important Are the Techniques?

There are women who have had natural childbirth most happily without any formal training at all. They have not used any special techniques, at least none that they were aware of using. There have been other women who have requested natural childbirth without the benefit of training and rehearsal for labor, and these women have run into difficulty in handling their labors. When this happens it causes an occasional doctor not experienced in prepared childbirth to feel that this new childbirth is not workable for the average woman, but works only for a rare, special kind of woman.

The techniques are not, of course, important in themselves except as they fulfill a need for comfort during childbirth. Some women don't have to use everything that they have learned, and they should not feel that they must use all that they have learned if they do not feel the need. They may feel fine with only some basic knowledge about childbirth and ways of handling the contractions.

Knowing the possibilities and the reasoning behind what is taught helps to build confidence in knowing what to do. Practicing the exercises and breathing helps women to feel comfortable with their bodies and to gain control over them during a time of stress as in labor. The techniques are really only common sense, but until recently most people have not thought about childbirth comfort in terms other than putting the woman into a confused stupor or interfering temporarily with the functioning of the nervous system by blocking sensation in the lower part of the body.

There is no controversy about the need for relaxation, pillows, and breathing in certain ways, but there is some controversy among doctors and others about the value of the physical conditioning exercises for birth, although everyone agrees that they increase comfort during pregnancy and speed the recovery from childbirth. They aid circulation, help to improve muscular control, and strengthen back and abdominal muscles, but *they do also get used during childbirth*. The pelvic rock may be used during labor for backache. Many women use the tailor sit during early labor or during transition and it helps to spread the thighs for delivery. The pelvic floor exercise is needed for birth because it gives control over the pelvic floor for delivery.

When selecting breathing methods to use for the first stage of labor before transition, among the techniques which have been found especially useful are: deep, slow breathing, then rib breathing when the level needs to be raised, and, finally, one of the high chest-breathing techniques such as Wright's "out" breathing, Kitzinger's "hummingbird" breathing or Bing's "Yankee Doodle" breathing.

III

Labor and Delivery

For husband and wife the labor and the delivery are the most important parts of the childbirth education program. They have learned the techniques, but how will they spend this day of birth? What will the day that their baby is born be like?

Going to the Hospital

Obstetricians tell their patients when to go to the hospital. The instructions given may vary depending on how far the patient lives from the hospital and whether this is the first or a subsequent baby. Typical instructions ask the patient to telephone if (1) regular contractions are occurring approximately ten minutes apart, or (2) a "pink show" is noticed as the mucous plug at the mouth of the uterus is dislodged, or (3) the bag of waters has broken, resulting in either a slow leak or in a rush of fluid.

Most people have heard about false labor contractions.

During the childbirth education class students have learned about these Braxton Hicks contractions and may have felt them in the later part of pregnancy. As the time for birth nears, Braxton Hicks contractions are distinguished from true labor contractions by the irregular time intervals between them, and by the fact that they have a tendency to disappear when the woman changes position. If she gets up or walks around they are likely to go away.

Labor contractions may start as a feeling of tightness in the abdomen, as pelvic pressure, or as backache. They usually occur at regular intervals, with the interval between gradually shortening. They do not go away when the woman changes position.

The bag of waters is the bag of colorless fluid which surrounds the developing baby in the uterus. At any time near birth it may break, or it may not break until labor is well advanced. The breaking of the bag of waters causes no discomfort. Women at home or, perhaps, out doing errands may not at first be certain of the source of the wetness. The liquid can be distinguished from urine by its odor because, of course, it does not smell like urine. If any odor is noticed, it will be mildly sweet. Doctors almost always prefer women to be in the hospital if the bag of waters has broken, even if there is no awareness yet of any labor contractions. Even if the bag of waters has broken there is no possibility of a "dry birth." The secreting cells keep on secreting, and, besides, the interior of the body is never dry.

The first symptoms of labor may be felt at any time. This may be after a heavy meal or early in the morning when the woman has had no food since the preceding day. Neither situation is to be recommended. Digestion comes to a halt when labor is well established, but an empty stomach for a long period of time before labor has actually begun may give rise to feelings of weakness and fatigue. Doctors sometimes allow a light meal before the woman comes to the hospital if she asks about this. Ginger ale, Jello, or tea with lots of sugar are most often recommended. When patients are admitted to the hospital they are asked what they last ate and when.

Just before labor begins women often have a burst of energy and do unnecessary chores instead of remaining rested. They may also stay up late because of the extra energy and the mounting feeling of excitement and anticipation. Sometimes, too, it is not easy to find a comfortable sleeping position, although the baby is often less active just before labor begins. Women should curb this impulse for activity if labor may be about to begin. They should not go into labor when they are either tired or very hungry.

During the prenatal period couples will have familiarized themselves with the route to the hospital and the entrance to be used. They will also, probably, have learned about admission procedures and toured the labor and delivery areas of the hospital as suggested in childbirth education classes.

Women are also encouraged to have their bags packed well ahead of time except for the husband's sandwich, which must be put in at the last minute. Hospital coffee shops may not be open all of the time, especially those run by volunteers. Also, many husbands do not want to leave their wives to find the coffee shop, especially as labor progresses and they get involved in the experience. Items to be taken to the hospital include the technique reminder sheet provided in most childbirth education classes, socks for cold feet, and a light robe so that the wife can get out of bed and still feel adequately covered. Hospital gowns are notoriously short. Other valuable items are Chapstick for dry lips and powder for back rubs and for the effleurage which may be used later in labor. Lollipops are often taken to provide sugar and moisture for dry mouths, but the ice chips provided by many hospitals are preferable. If glasses are worn they should be taken. They are useful in labor if she wants to read, and in delivery if the woman wishes to watch the birth in the delivery-room mirror. Bras will be needed for comfort during the early days after delivery. These should provide support and allow for expansion, whether or not breast feeding is planned. Sometimes these can be bought at the hospital. Women may wish to take their own sanitary belts and a small plastic bottle of liquid soap for light laundry.

Emergency Childbirth

Class couples often ask questions about what to do if something happens to prevent them from getting to the hospital on time, such as a flat tire or a snowstorm. Besides, babies sometimes arrive with very little warning. Not all classes offer information on emergency childbirth, but some knowledge can be reassuring. Rarely is it used.

If the wife realizes that birth is imminent, there is no need for panic and a wild, dangerous ride to the hospital. The husband should stop the car. His wife can either lie down on the back seat or she can remain sitting, but slumped down on the seat, to deliver over the edge of the seat with her husband to help her. He supports the baby's head as it emerges. A coat may be spread under the woman. The coat can be cleaned later more easily than can the car upholstery.

The woman should be helped to relax without being irritated by excessive attention. She should be kept warm but not too warm. She relaxes the vaginal area as taught in class. During delivery she does not push but does rapid shallow panting to help prevent tearing from a too rapid delivery. Any tears which do occur can be repaired later. The husband may support the lower edge of the birth canal gently to help avoid tearing, but he should not exert pressure on the baby's head, nor should he ever pull on the baby's head. The baby usually slides out easily without the need for any outside help.

Because the baby is slippery he must be held carefully, his head down or to the side to cough out any mucus which may be present in the throat. No rough treatment should be used to help the baby breathe. If there is any membrane covering the baby's face it must be removed. The cool air of the outside world acts as a stimulant to breathing, but as soon as the baby is breathing he should be wrapped.

Babies born in this way seldom have any problem breathing; however, the baby's back may be rubbed gently, and, if necessary, another aid to breathing can be used. Place one hand under the baby's hips and the other hand under his shoulders and head. Bring hands up together, bending baby's hips toward his shoulders to compress the stomach. Then straighten the baby's body. This activity performed twelve times per minute[1] produces movement of air in and out of lungs as in artificial respiration.

There should be no pulling on the cord to help expel the placenta, even if the placenta is not expelled spontaneously after a few minutes as generally happens. The baby remains attached to the other end of the cord. There is no rush about cutting the cord and it should be left uncut.

The baby should be placed at the mother's breast, taking care not to pull on the cord. The sucking of the baby helps the uterus to contract and reduces blood loss. If the baby swallows well there is no further need to worry about mucus in his mouth and throat. If there does seem to be mucus, the baby can be held with his head low and the mucus wiped out of his mouth very gently with a clean cloth. However, this is unlikely to be necessary. After the birth the husband resumes the drive to the hospital.

What to Expect from the Nurse in Labor and Delivery

In addition to her monitoring duties on pulse rates and other physical signs, the nurse in labor and delivery who understands prepared childbirth makes physical and emotional contact and offers a reassuring presence to the woman, or to the couple if the husband is present. She does not isolate the prepared couple but supports the relationship between husband and wife. She minimizes apprehension by giving information on progress of labor and reassurance as to its normality. Praise is offered when the woman uses her relaxation and breathing techniques effectively. Help is given her if she seems to be forgetting her techniques and becoming tense. The nurse also offers comfort measures as described below or helps the husband to provide them. She can help both prepared women and unprepared women in labor. The doctor is in charge of the patient, but the nurse makes certain that the patient gets the required care and support. In some ways she is actually in the role of a maternal model for the expectant couple.

Keane and Lesser[2] in their study found that women after delivery remembered the relationship provided by the nurse during labor as being most important to them. Although physical needs are usually seen as more acceptable needs, patients wanted someone to "stand by." Some nurses could create the feeling of "presence" even if not always in the room. It was also found that, when bodily needs were met promptly, pain relief and a renewed assurance of safety then occurred.

The nurse gives information on the progress of dilatation, but she cannot predict the length of labor. She does not say that the baby will not be born for several hours, that it will be "tonight" or "tomorrow," in order to avoid disappointing the patient in case the labor is a slow one. That kind of statement discourages the woman who may not be finding the contractions currently difficult but who does not care to think about their lasting indefinitely. It has often happened that the woman who has been told that she has several more hours to go has delivered within the next hour or less. The result can be loss of confidence in her attendants. Prepared women often do have shorter labors than unprepared, medicated patients.

A stream of words in a serene voice is reassuring. Praise is given for the ability to relax. As a contraction reaches its peak the woman is reminded by nurse or husband that it will be letting up soon.

The husband can be reminded by the nurse to breathe with his wife to help her maintain the rhythm if she seems to be losing control. If the husband or nurse does this breathing with her, emotional contact is also made so that she really feels the presence of those around her. She can also be helped to anticipate her contractions if a hand is placed on her abdomen. The abdomen hardens as the contraction builds. As the uterus begins to contract she must allow time for a stretch and the initial deep breath as she prepares to relax and breathe for the contraction.

Early Labor

Labor may begin with contractions at thirty-minute intervals and lasting, perhaps, twenty seconds, or it may start with other symptoms already mentioned. If labor starts at night, the woman is encouraged to sleep whether she is at home or in the hospital. This passes the time and allows her to be rested for the time later on when she will need to be alert. Despite the excitement of the baby's birth day, many women find that they can sleep.

The mouth of the uterus, the cervix, dilates at first slowly and then at an increasing rate during active labor and then again more slowly as it attains its maximum width of five fingers (10 centimeters). This will take usually a number of hours. This dilatation does not occur primarily because of the pressure of the baby's head on the cervix but is accomplished by the muscular action of the uterus.

Before labor begins the cervix has some thickness to it. When touched, it feels like the end of one's nose. As labor begins and the cervix is pulled back, the cervix becomes thinner until it is no thicker than the skin between the thumb and forefinger. This is called effacement. The cervix thins and it dilates. It may be thinning and dilating at the same time in early labor. If dilatation seems slow in early labor, there may still be progress in effacement. In fact, some work on effacement and dilatation has usually occurred even before the woman realizes she is in labor.

The amount of dilatation is usually determined by a finger inserted into the rectum. The cervix can be felt through the thin rectal wall. Sometimes the examinations are done vaginally. The woman receives no sensations from her cervix to tell her whether it is dilating or how much it has dilated, but experienced women can sometimes assess their own progress remarkably accurately.

Women who go into the hospital for induced labor know ahead of time when to go. Their labor is started by breaking the bag of waters and also, usually, by giving a synthetic hormone to start labor. An induced labor may be shorter, but unless there is a medical reason, the convenience of inductions is sometimes outweighed by the strong contractions which build up suddenly and which may last longer than in labors not artificially stimulated. Women and their doctors usually discuss this before going into the hospital.

If the woman enters the hospital during the day and her membranes are still intact, not yet ruptured, there is no need for her to be confined to bed. Walking may be helpful in early labor if she does not let herself get tired.

During early labor she will be interested in what is going on around her in the hospital. She will want companionship. The husband and wife may talk or play cards.

The husband times the contractions. The wife makes sure that she can relax in the way she has been taught, even is there is no need as yet. If she feels the excitement of the big day to such an extent that she finds it difficult to relax, she may take a mild tranquilizer in early labor.

Hospital procedures usually require an enema. This can increase the strength of the contractions, temporarily, to require the use of breathing and relaxing techniques.

Labor

Each labor is different, although each follows a certain progression. The dilatation stage is the longest. Two thirds of labor may be spent in reaching three fingers of dilatation. The dilatation cannot be hastened. The length of labor is related more to the strength and effectiveness of the contractions than to their frequency. This first stage is described as the one in which the woman "stays out of the way of her uterus" and lets dilatation take place unhindered. As previously described, the interval between the contractions will shorten and the intensity will increase, but the duration of the contractions will remain at about a minute. The peak of the intensity is usually at the middle of the contraction.

The untrained response to labor can be tight abdominal muscles and a jerky kind of breathing. Both of these responses interfere with the activity of the contracting uterus and cause increased pain as described in Chapter II.

Conscious relaxation is not started in early labor except to make certain that the woman can do it. She does not start it until she feels the need because it requires concentration. She does not use it between contractions as well as during contractions until later on in labor when there may be only a short interval between contractions.

Discomfort shows first in the face. If her toes are curled the woman is not relaxed. Tension tends to spread. The woman is encouraged to let her body mold into the bed, letting the bed totally support her. Her degree of relaxation can be checked as described in the section on relaxation techniques. Doing this will help her to become aware of any existing muscular tension.

The couple knows that each contraction is a step toward birth. One instructor tells her class couples to be patient with themselves. If they are not satisfied with the way they handle one contraction, they have plenty more to try! The woman takes each contraction as it comes. Between contractions she rests and thinks about how she will cope with the next contraction. Childbirth educators stress the necessity of "riding with" the contractions and "staying ahead" of them.

As labor becomes established, the woman's breathing as well as her degree of relaxation becomes important. Before each contraction she will take a quick, deep breath and relax all her muscles as she exhales. She then does the rhythmical breathing which increases in rate and shallowness as the contraction peaks and, as it subsides, breathes more deeply and slowly. The end of the contraction is always defined by another deep, cleansing breath. Nurses ask the woman what breathing method she has been taught, but conversation takes place between contractions, not during them. Breathing requires concentration and conversation interrupts the pattern of the breathing. Some women like to think about what is happening inside them during the contraction and to have a mental picture of the cervix opening.

Body position is important for comfort. As described earlier, the woman is never flat in bed with her abdomen pulled taut but has her head slightly raised, her knees and elbows slightly bent and supported by pillows. Her knees are rolled outward. A rolled towel or other device may be placed in the small of her back to prevent or relieve backache.

She should change position at least every two hours or

whenever the need is felt, using a position described in the section on comfort measures in Chapter II. If labor slows, the woman in labor may get up and walk around or, perhaps, shift to a side position. The side position may have been used for sleeping in the last months of pregnancy. It also allows a back rub to be given if desired.

Hospital personnel are definitely unaccustomed to women in labor getting out of bed to walk around! Nurses often feel more comfortable if patients stay in their beds, citing lack of space as a practical reason. The walk does not have to be one such as that depicted in one of the childbirth films showing a couple walking the sunny grounds of the hospital near the blue Pacific. Even a brief walk around the bed may be beneficial. It has been shown that fetal heart tones can be improved by maternal activity because a walk or a change of position stimulates the circulation.

If she gets confused on the breathing method or feels loss of control over her contractions, the woman may be told by those around her to sit straight up. The bed can be cranked up with a pillow in back of her head and under each knee. This can help her regain her alertness and feeling of control, and at the same time remove any back discomfort. This position is usually used for brief periods only.

Some women like to sit resting their arms on a table. The lower part of the body goes limp with the abdomen relaxed against the thighs. Women can read in this position between their contractions.

The bottom part of the top sheet on the bed should be untucked to avoid pinching the woman's toes and interfering with her relaxation.

Chilliness also interferes with relaxation. If the woman

feels cool she can be given a blanket and can wear socks. Heat applied to the abdomen can reduce soreness. If she feels warm, her face can be sponged with cool water.

Most women require ice chips for dry mouths because fluids are not given by mouth during labor even though there is no plan to use a gas anesthetic for delivery. Lollipops, a wet sponge, wet washcloth or paper towel are also used during labor, especially if no ice chips are available. Chapstick is often used on the lips. If a wet sponge or paper towel is used, the inside of the mouth is wiped, including the teeth. As one instructor says, "Nobody wants dry teeth." Placing the tongue on the roof of the mouth during mouth breathing is sometimes done to reduce dryness of the mouth. The routine use of intravenous fluids, without special reason, is annoying and unnecessary.

During labor the wife does not hold the husband's hand because if she is squeezing she is not relaxing. He may hold her hand if she wishes physical contact.

She should get up every two hours to empty her bladder even if she does not feel the need. Discomfort is associated with bladder fullness, even though during labor she may be unaware of the source of the discomfort and feel no urge to void. The bladder does accumulate urine even though the woman is not drinking fluids. A distended bladder takes up space in the abdominal cavity and interferes with labor contractions.

Effleurage as described in Chapter II can be done by the woman herself or by her husband. If pain is felt in the legs they should be rubbed firmly by the husband or nurse.

Abdominal lifting is another comfort measure which can be done by the husband. Many women like this, but it is strenuous for those who attend them. The fingers are hooked under the ribs and the distended abdomen is lifted with each contraction. It is started as the contraction starts. As the woman inhales the baby is lifted, thus removing the pressure of the uterus on the back. The woman must not arch her back during this procedure but must let the person helping her do the work.

During labor the woman concentrates on what she is doing, knowing that if there is any medical problem she will be told and that the obstetrician and staff are prepared to handle it.

The obstetrician may rupture the membranes surrounding the baby at some time during the course of the labor, a procedure which causes no discomfort at all to the woman. If this is done at any time after 3 fingers dilatation the labor can be expected to move rapidly. If the water breaks early, the increased intensity of the contractions is usually temporary.

If, near the end of the dilatation stage, the woman feels that she is losing control of her labor and that the techniques are not working well for her, she is probably entering transition.

Transition

Transition is the most difficult part of the labor, but it is also the shortest. The coping mechanisms which have been workable before transition are suddenly found to be no longer adequate. If the woman remembers her training she will not be surprised if these contractions last as long as seventy-five seconds. Occasionally there seems to be a double-header when the contractions come so close together that they almost blend into one. There may be as little as thirty seconds between contractions, but this interval of rest is important.

New and unfamiliar symptoms such as nausea, chills, trembling of the thighs, and changes in mood may be observed. There is often a panicky feeling of being trapped as she moves toward the climax of birth. There is a final awareness that a baby is going to arrive and that there is no turning back now. During this time of transition the body is preparing for the next stage, that of moving the baby out of the uterus into the birth canal, and the symptoms are related to this imminent change. They are temporary.

If the woman needs to vomit during transition and there is no pan available, she should vomit on the floor. Otherwise the bed sheets will have to be changed. If there should be any nausea, it can often be relieved by using slow, controlled breathing temporarily instead of the more rapid types usually used in transition.

She has no wish for non-essential conversation. She may become irritable if touched or examined. But she does want someone with her, and she should never be left alone at this time, not even to get medication. Medication is not useful at this late stage anyway. It would not work in time to relieve the discomfort of this stage and would only make her tired and sleepy for the delivery. Instead, she needs someone to sit with her, work with her, breathe with her.

The breathing techniques are of the greatest help during transition. The woman uses whatever techniques she has chosen to learn and practice. She may count, mouth words, tap out a rhythm on her thigh to satisfy her need for distraction and activity in ways which will not interfere with the work of the uterus. The breathing methods used at this time give a continuous but very slight movement of the diaphragm.

Many women do not want to lie down during this stage unless they are in the side position. Some women prefer to be more or less sitting during the entire labor because they feel more comfortable and more in control of their situation in this way. The body positions used during transition are any of those which have been described. More than one may have to be tried to see which one helps. The woman may need reminders of what positions to try. Some women tend to want to remain motionless at this time, fearing that they will experience pain if they move. A favorite position is that of sitting up almost at right angles in a cross-legged position with the knees resting on pillows.

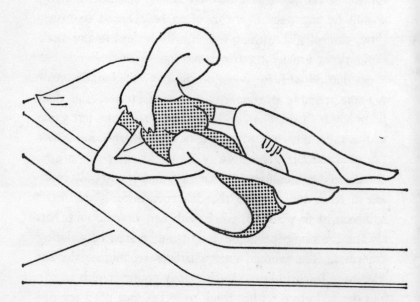

The hospital bed is raised all the way up for back support. Two overlapping pillows are placed behind her head and shoulders for a "shingle" effect. She may want to get up on all fours.

The up-on-all fours position is still an unusual sight in a hospital labor room, but it is becoming more popular, especially if the other positions do not offer enough help. This position has also been found useful in helping to rotate the baby's head to an anterior position if it is not already in this position, although it usually is. If the baby is born in the usual face-down position, the back of his head (the occiput) will be toward the front part (anterior) of his mother's body. This is the easiest position for birth and almost all babies are born in this position. If the baby happens to be in the position where he will deliver face up, he may rotate himself to a face-down position or, rather, be rotated by the forces in the mother's body because the baby is simply a passenger. If this does not occur, the doctor may rotate the baby so that he will not arrive "sunny side up." But, although turning over and getting up on the hands and knees does act to help rotate a posterior head, this activity is a comfort measure whatever the baby's position. A gentle pelvic rock done at the same time feels good and gives additional relief, especially because labor is so often felt in the back during transition.

Any of the comfort measures previously described for use in labor can also be used during transition.

The urge to push is often beginning to be felt, but not always. To prevent wasting energy and possible damage to the cervix, the trained woman resists the urge by doing shallow blowing.

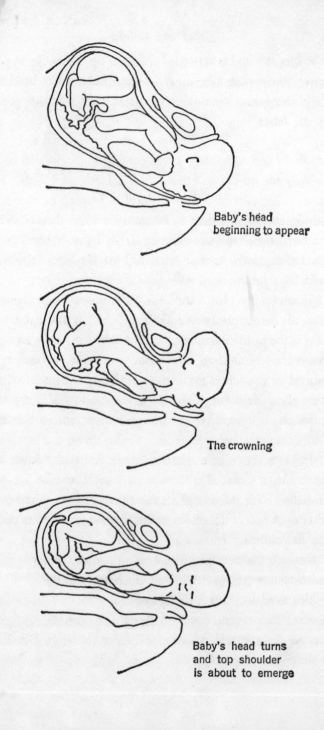

Baby's head beginning to appear

The crowning

Baby's head turns and top shoulder is about to emerge

When the dilatation stage is completed the woman feels better. She gets a chance to rest and catch her breath before the pushing stage, the most comfortable and satisfying part of the labor.

Delivery

During the second stage of labor the baby is moved down the birth canal toward delivery. This is made possible by the action of the uterus aided by the diaphragm, the abdominal muscles, and the respiratory muscles.

As the couple has learned to expect from the preparation, the contractions are less frequent and do not last as long as they did during transition. They also give a bearing-down kind of feeling. There may be only a few of these contractions or they may continue for about an hour, but there is no longer any need to remain relaxed during these contractions except for the perineal relaxation in the birth area.

The first sign of the approaching delivery stage may be a catch in her breathing. Or she may say that she needs to push and ask if she should do this. If she is fully dilated, and there is no rim or lip of the cervix left, she will be told that she can push.

Women often dislike the rushed move from the labor room to the delivery room at this time, but rarely are facilities available which allow women to labor and deliver in the same room. Hospital people are usually very distressed at the possibility of the baby arriving in bed. Even if they have been calm and almost lackadaisical during the labor, they become very active as delivery nears. Occasionally at this time the woman is alone, briefly, as the husband goes to get the nurse, who then goes to call the obstetrician. The woman must keep her cool and remember her training.

When hospital staff have determined that delivery is imminent, the woman is quickly wheeled from the labor room to the delivery room. She must then, at this awkward time just before birth, be transferred to the delivery table. She can climb onto the delivery table herself. There is no need to lift her and being lifted can be uncomfortable. She takes her pillows with her.

With each contraction the baby's head comes down and then recedes somewhat as the wave of the contraction subsides, but the head does not recede to the place where it was when the contraction started.

The untrained or unconscious woman may arch her back, raise her buttocks off the table, and throw her head back. She often pushes with little air in her lungs so that the diaphragm is not being used effectively to aid expulsion. She may also clamp down with her vaginal muscles to interfere with the delivery. In addition, the untrained or anesthetized woman usually delivers in the lithotomy position flat on her back with her legs raised in stirrups. This position has its advantages for gynecological surgery or anesthetized mothers, but because of the angle of the vagina, it actually forces the woman to push the baby uphill. It is also thought by some to increase the need for routine episiotomy besides causing difficulty in pushing.

Doctors and nurses do not place prepared women in the lithotomy position. If stirrups are used at all, they are placed low. The prepared woman delivers in a semi-propped position with her back curved, her head and shoulders supported by one or two pillows or by her husband's arm under her shoulders. The nurse is on one side of her and the husband on the other. Her head is forward and her knees drawn up. She can then take her deep inspiration breaths and bear down. It feels good to follow the urge to push.

During the delivery stage the activity of those around her is important to the woman. She needs to feel their encouragement and their response to the forces which are occurring within her. When the baby's head can be seen she is told, and she is kept informed of the progress as more of the baby's head can be seen. She is coached through every contraction by the team around her, the obstetrician, the nurse, and the husband. She does not have to start pushing with the very beginning of the contraction but can add her voluntary efforts a few seconds after the contraction has begun. She needs help with the timing and getting into position.

The trained woman herself can usually judge how hard she needs to push until the actual time of delivery when the obstetrician must tell her. If, at the beginning of the pushing stage, she finds that it hurts to push, she realizes that her body is not quite ready, and she waits for a few minutes. She then tries again. Pushing should not be very forceful until her body tells her that she needs to push harder. Aggressive pushing can be a mistake. Speed is not the criterion. She pushes as hard as she needs to in order to "push the discomfort away," and she finds that she does know how hard to push even though childbirth is a new experience for her.

Between contractions she lies back and rests from the exertion. She may talk or ask questions.

As delivery nears, the woman pushes less hard. The perineum thins gradually. It tends to lose feeling and if a laceration were to occur she might not be aware of it. The obstetrician at the foot of the table can see the progress. He gives directions on when to push and how hard to push. He also tells the woman when she should not push at all. The goal is a smooth, controlled delivery. The baby must not be ejected with insensitive force. When the crown of the head can be seen, the next contraction will probably deliver the head. The woman then holds back slightly, does her panting breathing, and should be told by her obstetrician not to push at all to make the delivery gentle on the perineum and on the baby's head. The force exerted by the uterus alone is sufficient. The woman can stop pushing even though the urge to push is strong.

An episiotomy is usually done and is thought beneficial for many. Some controversy surrounds the practice, which is done almost routinely in the United States, especially because women often find the healing very painful. In a book written for parents the comment is made that

> In cases where an episiotomy is not necessary, it is usually because the mother in labor tends to balance her bearing-down efforts against the discomfort produced by the stretching of the vagina and adjacent tissues. This balancing may ensure a gradual stretching of the vagina so that a small or normal-sized baby can pass through the birth canal without requiring additional space. This may be true of a woman having either a first or subsequent baby. However, once an episiotomy has been performed on a mother, most doctors prefer to repeat it when her succeeding babies are born.[3]

Most doctors in the United States feel more certain that the perineal tone will be maintained if episiotomies are performed, and most prepared women expect to have this procedure. There is no evidence from studies that episiotomies prevent the need for gynecological repair later on, but the routine episiotomy is based on this assumption. Therefore, even though there may not appear to be a need for the procedure, it is usually done anyway. The incision affects only the external tissues. For the prepared woman the obstetrician may make only a small cut.

As the baby arrives face down and turns his head to the side his eyes and mouth are usually open. There may be another contraction for the shoulders and body. The mother feels relief from the pressures she has experienced, and also an emotional excitement as she hears the first cry. She rises up on her elbows to see the child she and her husband have produced. She looks for response and reassurance from those around her.

The new mother may be handed the baby even before the cord is cut. The cord is 20 to 40 inches long. It is stiff like a garden hose from the hydrostatic pressure within it and is therefore not easily knotted. It contains no pain fibers. Preferably, the cord is not cut immediately. The cord blood belongs to the baby, and if the obstetrician waits until it stops pulsating before cutting it, the baby receives as much as 100 cc. of blood volume.

Professional responsibilities of nurse and obstetrician take most of their attention. The baby's skin may be wiped off. He is wrapped and silver nitrate is put into his eyes. If state regulations have been changed to allow the use of antibiotic ointment, this is used instead of the silver nitrate, which reddens the eyes.

The obstetrician waits a few minutes for the placenta to deliver. The delivery of the placenta is called the third stage of labor. The mother may push once more for the placenta but seldom feels any discomfort as it delivers spontaneously. Nourishment and oxygen have passed through the placenta during pregnancy even though the blood of mother and baby have not mixed. The mother can be shown the placenta if she wishes. It is the size of a small pie and is an iridescent red in color. It is a unique and complex organ from which hormones are extracted commercially.

The obstetrician next busies himself with sewing up the episiotomy.

The new mother may have to ask for her baby if he is not given to her. She may nurse her baby on the delivery table or perhaps spend a few minutes with the baby first before trying to nurse. The father may hold the baby too. It is important that new parents have their first meeting with their baby promptly. Each baby is different right from the beginning and has his own ways of responding.

The new mother feels well. She could get up and walk off the delivery table. She is thirsty and may get a drink even in the delivery room. She has feelings of release and accomplishment. She is "high" and, often, so is the father. She is not ready to fall asleep immediately after giving birth. Neither does she want to be left by herself. She wants to see the new baby, to talk and to unwind.

She does not stay in the delivery room very long but is usually moved to a recovery room. Medicated and anesthetized mothers may spend several hours there before going back to their rooms, but lightly medicated or unmedicated women who have not had anesthesia do not usually lie in the recovery room very long. The time spent in the recovery room depends on the condition of the mother, hospital policy, and on when there is someone available to move her back to her room.

IV

Drugs and Anesthesia

The subject of the painkillers used in childbirth is an almost total mystery to most people. They know very little about medication (drugs) and anesthesia. The unprepared woman who asks to be "knocked out" often believes, mistakenly, that she will be anesthetized for the whole labor and delivery. She does not know the difference between the drugs given to relieve pain in labor and the anesthetic given for the delivery. Women who have not had preparation for childbirth have usually had their babies without knowing why they were awake, if they were awake, or when or if they would later be unconscious. Accurate information for parents is difficult to obtain, but it is given in childbirth classes.

Before childbirth education came onto the scene it was usually thought a favor to women to give them everything possible in the way of drugs within the limits of safety, even though the limits of safety are still not entirely known. There is no ideal drug or anesthetic to produce sleep or relieve pain which does not also have other effects on the mother's body. Most drugs and the inhalation gas type of anesthesia have an obvious effect on newborns. Most of the substances used are a great help when needed, but their effects cannot be disregarded[1] and there is a difference between seeing them as something to be routinely administered to all patients and seeing them as valuable tools to be used when needed.

The use of medication alone for the unprepared woman cannot be expected to relieve all pain, especially if the woman is tense and afraid. If, later on, she does not recall pain or has no recollection of the labor and delivery, she probably had an amnesic drug which keeps her from remembering. For the prepared woman who uses the relaxation and breathing techniques the situation is entirely different. She knows very well what is happening and she often needs no drugs or anesthesia at all.

The obstetrician writes the orders for drugs and anesthesia. Why do parents need the information? Parents desiring a cooperating, participating childbirth experience certainly do need some basic orientation. The obstetrician wants to know the kind of childbirth experience which the woman desires. She cannot discuss her needs intelligently without some knowledge of the several ways of achieving pain relief. Obstetricians may or may not explain pharmacological pain relief to their patients, but the time factor usually leaves many questions unanswered. Patients will ask more useful questions if they have some background knowledge. Also, patients feel to an increasing degree entitled to know what is being given them and to make choices where appropriate.

Obstetricians will not want to commit themselves in the office ahead of time to a decision on exactly how they will handle a given situation, but if parents and obstetrician understand each other's feelings, dissatisfaction later on is more likely to be avoided. Women like to feel that there is a kind of partnership between them and their obstetricians. They do not want to feel, as one patient said, like an adversary to be kept under restraint, a feeling which can be reinforced if the sides of the bed are raised. Husbands and wives ask, "What do you like to give if it is hard to relax in early labor?" or "How do you feel about the routine use of anesthesia for delivery?" They also say that they don't want medication in place of emotional support, or so much medication that it will interfere with the use of the techniques they have learned. If they have the typical dose of a medication they cannot possibly concentrate adequately on breathing and relaxing, or even remember what they have learned. Medication does not have to be an "either or" situation in which the patient is either totally medicated or has "natural" childbirth. Nor do firm decisions about medication have to be made at six weeks of pregnancy during the first office visit. The woman knows what she needs when the time comes if she is getting adequate help and support and has had preparation for childbirth. Doctors can leave orders for medication to be given at the patient's request, and will usually do so if there has been doctor-patient communication ahead of time. Medication and anesthesia are not given to promote health but to relieve suffering and to allow obstetric interference if there is a need for it.

Anesthesia may be given by the obstetrician or a nurse-anesthetist, but there is another person who may have a role in the delivery. He is the anesthesiologist. The patient meets him for the first time in early labor when he enters her room to discuss her preference for anesthesia at the time of delivery. There is not much opportunity for women to learn about anesthesia at this time. Anesthesiologists are able to allow unprepared women to be awake with a caudal or epidural instead of the medication and spinals so typically used for unprepared women. Anesthesiologists have also been understanding of women's desire for prepared childbirth without routine anesthesia and are willing to stand by in case they are needed.

Besides providing techniques for pain relief, childbirth education instruction produces certain attitudes and results. Knowledge about childbirth processes helps women to achieve confidence and relaxation, to avoid fear, tension, and the inability to cooperate. The knowledge that medication is available can help relaxation because women can relax much more easily if they know something about the available drugs and their effects. Most women do not mind some pain if the labor is progressing well. Since the contractions do not usually last more than a minute, women often prefer to feel some pain instead of trying to cope with contractions under the influence of drugs which make it difficult to concentrate on the task at hand. If the doctor wishes to speed labor by using a synthetic hormone similar to oxytocin, the body hormone associated with uterine contraction, the woman needs to know that the contractions will be both stronger and longer in duration for a while. If she does not know this she may become frightened.

The ways in which medication is used can alter markedly the normal childbirth experience for parents. This fact offers another reason for parents to have some knowledge and choices. For instance, hospitals may have regulations about husbands staying with medicated wives. If the wife is awake and relatively comfortable, the couple can share the birth experience. If the wife receives enough medication to prevent her from being in control of her mind and body, her husband may have to leave because she is not really "there." She may wake later to find him gone.

Women used to be told by nurses that they should take the medication early because, later on, it would be too late. This was said because (1) it is not wise to have a substantial amount of a drug which depresses respiration in the mother's body at the time of delivery, when it can affect the baby's ability to breathe, and (2) the drug might make her too sleepy to push. However, it was found that if the time is "too late" because she is at or near transition and delivery, she doesn't need a drug, not even a small dose.

Medication

Medication, not anesthesia, is given during labor. As described in Chapter I, medication (analgesia) is used to raise the threshold of pain or to induce sleep. Anesthesia, on the other hand, blocks consciousness or it blocks sensation. The woman cannot be anesthetized for the long hours required for the cervix to dilate, and anesthesia would slow or halt labor. However, there are regional block anesthetics which can be used during the dilatation stage, but the regional block does tend to slow labor.

Obstetricians usually have their favorite medications. A *narcotic* such as demerol is commonly used, or a short-acting synthetic narcotic such as nisentil. Many obstetricians use nisentil very successfully for prepared patients to help them relax yet remain in control of their labors. More than a minimum dose of demerol, for example, can cause dizziness, sleepiness, and difficulty in concentration for the mother who wants a conscious, participating birth. Dosages are not taught in childbirth classes, but hospitals have found a dose of demerol as small as 25 mg. to be effective. This is one fourth of a typical dose of demerol. How much medication is "too much" depends on the drug used, on the woman, her degree of relaxation, and on other medication she may have had. A frightened woman requires a larger dose than a relaxed woman.

Narcotics do pass through the placenta to the baby. Respiratory depression in the newborn can result. Sometimes narcotic antagonists are used to combat the depressive effects of a narcotic.

Barbiturates are another type of medication frequently used in combination with a narcotic, especially for untrained women. These substances act by inducing sleep. Seconal has often been used. Nembutal is another barbiturate used during labor. Barbiturates and narcotics, in dosages used for childbirth, do not ordinarily produce long periods of unconsciousness, especially during the daytime. The barbiturates have little effect on pain in the dosages used, but they do have a sedative effect. Seconal reaches the baby in about one minute. Newborns are sensitive to barbiturates given to the mother during labor, and the effects can last several days. Barbiturates are not given close to the time of delivery when it is important that the baby breathe promptly.

Tranquilizers are the other major group of drugs used during labor. These drugs may act as synergists, meaning that they work with other drugs to increase their effectiveness.

Heavily medicated women who have had substantial

doses of one, two, or three drugs may have labor slowed besides losing the ability to cooperate with the labor and the doctor's directives. They may be given an oxytocic drug to stimulate labor.

Scopolamine is the *amnesic* drug given to women who expect to "sleep" through the birth. Its effects are described in Chapter I. It does not remove pain but acts to remove memory. It is a hallucinogen and causes the irrational behavior so often seen in labor rooms, and it also encourages fears about childbirth for all who witness its effects unless they learn about it before going into labor themselves. It is not used for prepared women.

Scopolamine is also a drying agent and therefore doctors who plan to use inhalation gas anesthesia sometimes say that they like to use scopolamine for this reason. They want a dry mouth and throat before giving this anesthesia. However, not all doctors feel that this drying is necessary and may use atropine if they want to use anything at all before giving gas. Atropine is not a hallucinogen.

Anesthesia

Anesthesia for childbirth may be a simple shot of novocain in the perineum for the episiotomy stitches or the women may be totally unconscious. Anesthesia is usually given during the second, or delivery, stage of labor when the baby is being pushed down the birth canal. It can be one of two types, general or conduction anesthesia. General anesthesia, or inhalation anesthesia, as it may also be called, consists of a gas which is inhaled to cause loss of consciousness. Conduction anesthesia, such as spinal or epidural, blocks nerve impulses. Sensation is blocked and sometimes the ability to move the legs is temporarily lost, as with a spinal, but consciousness remains.

Usually, but not always, forceps must be used for an anesthetized delivery. Anesthesia interferes with uterine contraction and with the ability or urge to bear down to push out the baby. Because the pushing stage is a more comfortable stage than the dilatation stage, women who do not know that this is so sometimes give all the credit for pain relief to the anesthesia. However, anesthesia is very effective in providing pain relief whether or not the woman has been trained or educated for birth.

Anesthesia has traditionally been given for delivery as part of the obstetrical services to patients, even if little medication was used during labor. With the advent of women educated for childbirth there has been improved understanding of women's ability to control the pushing stage if taught, and greater understanding that there is little pain in the second stage.

General Anesthesia

General or inhalation anesthesia, consisting of one of several gas or gas-oxygen combinations, is a fast-acting anesthesia which takes effect almost immediately. It is used when the obstetrician wants anesthesia quickly. The stomach must be empty when it is given or there may be nausea and inhalation of food particles. If the woman does have food in her stomach another type of anesthesia must be used.

General anesthesia reduces the amount of oxygen reaching the baby's brain and tissues. Too much anesthesia can interfere with his ability to breathe after birth. About two minutes is required for the gas to reach the baby after it is given to the mother.

This anesthesia causes relaxation of the uterine muscle. The gas is used for a brief period of time, only a few minutes. The woman is unconscious for the birth. Sometimes whiffs are given at the peak of the contraction to take the edge off any discomfort, the woman regaining consciousness between contractions.

General anesthesia is used less often now. It has been largely replaced by the conduction anesthesias, which are safer and which allow the woman to remain conscious. General anesthesia is also associated with more blood loss than are the conduction anesthesias, but both types are associated with more blood loss after delivery than occurs in an unanesthetized delivery, in which there is usually very little blood loss.

Conduction Anesthesia

Conduction anesthesia is regional anesthesia in which a substance such as xylocaine or novocain is injected into the body at a location which will block the transmission of nerve impulses to the brain. The nerves affected depend on the location of the blockade. A skilled anesthetist is required to administer the anesthesia. The woman remains awake and the anesthesia does not cause respiratory depression in the baby. Numbness occurs in the lower part of the body, but the woman can move her legs unless a spinal has been given. The urge to bear down is a reflex urge which is inhibited by regional anesthesia, even by the pudendal block. This is because the sensory nerve impulses, which would normally travel from the pelvic area to the spinal cord and from there up to the brain, are blocked. Without these impulses the reflex urge to bear down does not occur even though the woman can push when told to. When the blockade is higher on the body, as with a spinal, not only are the sensory nerve impulses blocked but also many of the motor impulses coming from the brain to the muscles. This is why she cannot move her legs.

Spinal Anesthesia

The injection is given into the spinal fluid after the woman has passed through the transition stage of labor. It may be given when the obstetrician can see a small patch of the baby's head, about the size of a fifty-cent piece, at the height of the contraction. If given earlier it would interfere with the labor. It does act to stop labor, therefore requiring a forceps delivery in most cases. A spinal is sometimes given if the woman is too tired to push for some reason, or if she is not relaxing the pelvic floor muscles adequately. It may be given if the delivery is delayed and the doctor wants to "go in after the baby." It may be given for the last contraction when the head is on the perineum to give perineal relaxation. Spinals are also used to delay the delivery, as well as to hasten it, depending on the desire of the obstetrician.

The effect of the spinal is to relax the uterus, although not as much as does general anesthesia. There is numbness below the spot where the spinal was given. The abdomen hardens during contractions, showing that the uterus is still contracting, but the contractions do not have force and downward pressure. Because the control over the abdominal muscles is reduced, the woman's ability to bear down is reduced, but she can bear down as long as she retains the power over her diaphragm, upper abdominal muscles, the muscles around her ribs, and other muscles of respiration.

Sometimes there is a temporary drop in blood pressure, but spinals have no effect on the infant unless the decreased blood pressure interferes with the circulation to the uterus. Vasopressor substances are sometimes used to counteract the blood-pressure drop if necessary. They act to raise the blood pressure, the assumption being that blood flow to the uterus will also be increased.

When the spinal is given the woman feels only a pinprick. She lies on her side with knees drawn up and head forward to give maximum space between the vertebrae.

The spinal headaches, lasting hours or even days, seldom occur now that finer-gauge needles are used and there is, therefore, less leakage of spinal fluid.

Saddle Block

The saddle block is often called a "little spinal." It is a low spinal given by needle with the woman in a sitting position. It is put in between contractions. It is not given to a hysterical patient or one with chronic back problems. Although constant attendance of the patient is needed, the safety factor is increased because less quantity of the drug is needed and the extent of the anesthesia is less. The blood pressure can be lowered, however, as with a spinal.

The area of anesthesia resembles that of the caudal, but the saddle block is easier to give and more precise. It is given with the woman sitting up with her head forward. She feels only a pinprick. It anesthetizes the part of the body which would touch a saddle if riding a horse, and the perineum, vulva, and vagina. It relaxes the perineum and gives partial anesthesia of the legs.

Caudal Anesthesia

Caudal anesthesia is put into the low back outside the spinal canal at the tail of the spine. It does not mix with the spinal fluid. It anesthetizes the sensory nerves but has almost no effect on motor nerves so the woman can move. It takes ten to twenty minutes to give, and the catheter remains in place, allowing more anesthesia to be given as needed.

No headaches result from caudals. They can be given earlier than the spinals because they diminish the contractions only slightly. For a first baby the cervical dilatation should be about four fingers (or 8 cm.).

Epidural Anesthesia

Epidural anesthesia is continuous like the continuous caudal, and is similar to the caudal. It is useful for women who wish to be awake but who have not had training for childbirth. A very small polyethylene tube is placed in the back a little higher than for the caudal and remains there until after the delivery. The anesthetic substance bathes the nerve endings but does not mix with the spinal fluid. Like the caudal, it may be given at about four fingers' dilatation. It may be helpful for transition, but does not always help with transition. Sometimes it is given earlier than four fingers' dilatation if the head is really down in the pelvis. Women have complained about discomfort when it is given even though expert technique is used in inserting it. Forceps are used for delivery.

Epidurals are expensive because they require skill and constant observation. They can also slow labor and cause a drop in blood pressure.

Paracervical Anesthesia

Paracervicals and pudendals are local anesthesias. The paracervical is given by inserting the needle through the vagina into the cervix. The effect lasts about an hour and can be renewed by another injection if needed. It is given early enough in labor so that the cervix can still be found. The injection is given in several places in the cervix with the needle slanted away from the baby's head.

It is a good anesthesia for a tight cervix which is not dilating well. Its only disadvantage is that sometimes the baby's heart slows markedly after the injections. Smaller doses may help prevent this undesirable effect.

Pudendal Anesthesia

Xylocaine is injected into the pudendal nerve. The injection is given through the buttocks aimed toward the pelvic bones on each side. It gives outlet anesthesia. The mother does not feel the baby coming out. She must be coached when to push because she does not feel the desire to do so.

"Nature's Anesthesia"

Because the gradual descent of the baby's head often removes much of the sensory awareness in the pelvic area, episiotomies have even been done without pain to the mother. They have also been repaired after delivery, using "nature's anesthesia" if they can be done quickly before the effect wears off. There is no real benefit from attempting this. A little novocain in the perineum for the episiotomy is given to prepared women.

A Final Word on Drugs and Anesthesia

Greenhill[2] points out that "the pain-relieving drugs used during labor are among the most powerful substances known in pharmacology." Brazelton continues his research and Kron has been another researcher on obstetric sedation. The temporary effects of medication on mother and baby are obviously better known than are the long-term effects. In 1969 a paper presented at a meeting in Santa Monica to the Society for Research in Child Development stated that there was a perceptible effect on the newborn's response to a conditioned stimulus which could still be seen in one-month-old babies whose mothers had been drugged at birth.

In June of 1970 the Society for Research in Child Development published a monograph[3] on the effects of obstetric medication on the fetus and infant. The International Childbirth Education Association summarized this monograph in its November–December 1970 *Bulletin*, saying that "the monograph's twelve page bibliography extensively documents the fact that virtually all obstetric medications—amnesics, analgesia and anesthetics including the medication used for caudal, epidural, paracervical and pudendal anesthesia—rapidly cross the placental barrier and enter the fetal blood supply within a short time of their administration to the mother." It has long been known that inhalation anesthesia and analgesic drugs cross the placental barrier, but this study refutes the accepted view that scopolamine and conduction anesthesias have no direct effect on the baby.

Drugs and anesthesia *are* needed in obstetrics, but they do not need to be given just because women are afraid of childbirth. Also, they do not need to be given in doses larger than necessary to do the job they are intended to do, nor should they replace teaching women about childbirth.

V

FATHER, MOTHER, AND BABY

After the delivery has been accomplished, the postpartum and newborn periods begin simultaneously. Both mother and baby move into a new stage of the life cycle. The new father does too.

The new childbirth has brought changes in attitudes and in practices. It has been found that there is no need to make the introduction to parenthood as emotionally sterile as is the physical plant of the hospital. When mothers were groggy with anesthesia and their husbands were either at home or in the hospital waiting room, there seemed to be nothing unusual about the custom of trundling the baby out of the delivery room and down to the nursery without either parent having more than a brief glimpse of their new child on the way by, if that. The feeling was that the primary need of mother and baby was that of rest. Mother and baby could meet later when both were more rested. If the mother protested, she might even be given a tranquilizer to quiet her. The same feeling prevailed about food. Nourishment came after rest and recovery from anesthesia, regardless of when the mother had her last meal. These customs no longer made sense when mothers were wide awake and fathers were present for birth.

The awake woman who has had prepared childbirth does not make negative comments about her baby or say that she would rather see the baby later. If she has not had medication or has had very little, she is prepared to make a response to the baby, a response which is thwarted if the baby goes directly to the nursery. It is a handicap to the establishment of the parent-child bond if the couple does not share with each other the first meeting with their child. The baby belongs to the couple, not to the hospital, the grandparents, or the in-laws. The meeting does not have to be long if nurses are busy. Even a minute or two can be a help.

The baby is awake for a while after birth and he needs the physical contact of being held before being wheeled down to be added to the row of cribs in the nursery. Gentle handling helps to stimulate his breathing and circulation.

The Baby

The newborn is handled gently. There is no need to prove how tough he is. As he is born the pressures on his body are suddenly released. He is in a bright, dry, and cool environment. His circulation changes to send blood through his lungs. He must now take his first breath. Sometimes he takes his first breath before he is completely born, especially if he has not received medication. Before birth his lungs were squeezed up like a sponge.[1] After the separation of the placenta from the uterus, during or shortly after birth, the baby lacks an oxygen supply even though his mother's oxygen continues to go to him until the cord becomes white if the cord is not cut immediately. As the baby loses his oxygen supply from his mother, the lack of oxygen causes signals to pour up to the gasping part of the brain. The muscle walls of the cord shut down on the baby's blood, preventing it from going back into the cord. The heart valves tend to close, causing blood to be pumped through the lungs. The pressure of the changed circulation further closes the heart valves. The signals to the brain cause the baby's ribs to expand, allowing air to enter the lungs for the first time. The expansion of the ribs now causes signals to go to the respiratory center of the brain to stimulate expiration. The vocal cords then tighten, and with the first expiratory breath comes the infant's well-known first cry.

The cord is cut and tied, but a little bit of it, the stump, is left on the baby. It will dry up, turn black, and drop off in a few days.

Of course, the newborn's face and body structure are different from what they will be later. The nose is flatter and the chin recedes. The head is large. The baby's appearance changes minute by minute as his color changes from blue to purplish to pink. The hands and feet remain purplish longest. As the hours pass his skin becomes less wrinkled.

To allay possible unnecessary worries about their baby's safe arrival, parents need to know that new babies have some or all of the following: forceps marks over the cheekbones if forceps have been used, white spots on the skin from plugged sweat glands, or maybe some red spots on the skin which have sometimes been called "stork bites." The skin is very thin and the small blood capillaries may be visible, especially on the eyelids or back of the neck. There may have been molding of the head as it passed through the bony pelvis and birth canal, causing the back of the head to be more prominent than it will be shortly. There can be some swelling of a spot on the top of the head where it was pushed against the cervix with each contraction. This molding and swelling are possible because the bones in the head are still soft and have spaces between them. Temporary swelling of the sex organs may occur because of the mother's hormones. Blood on the scalp can come from the mother's episiotomy as he was delivered. All of these characteristics of the newborn are temporary.

If silver nitrate rather than antibiotic ointment is used for the baby's eyes after delivery, the eyes may look red and puffy for a couple of days as a result of the silver nitrate. The baby's first bowel movement after birth will be black and tarry. It is called meconium and was present in the intestines before birth. On the third day after birth some babies have a temporary jaundice as the liver begins to function. Vitamin K given routinely at the time of birth may also promote some jaundice temporarily. It is given to promote the clotting ability of the baby's blood, especially if a circumcision is to be done. After a few days the baby swallows enough bacteria to be able to manufacture his own vitamin K in his intestines.

The baby's hearing at birth is good. He heard sounds in his mother's body, including her heartbeat before he was born. He also heard some sounds from the outside world. At birth he sees better than was formerly thought although he must learn to use his eyes together. Even before he was born he could see light dimly through his mother's abdomen if she stood in bright sunlight.

The healthy baby's major needs from those who care for him are not complicated. Instead of a period of enforced isolation without human contact, he needs sucking, holding, feeding, an occasional change of sleeping position, diaper changes, and warmth from those who care for him.

Circumcision on the boy baby is done by the obstetrician a few days after birth. Parent permission is required. Although there is still some controversy about this procedure it is now done almost routinely in the United States. If parents have any doubts, they might want to discuss them with a pediatrician besides talking with the obstetrician. Parents often ask if an anesthetic is given. The answer is generally no, although wine, whiskey, or sugar water have been given to babies.

The Mother

Her first needs are (1) meeting the baby and feeding it if she wishes; (2) talking with her husband as she unwinds from the childbirth experience; (3) nourishment; and (4) rest or sleep, especially if the baby was born during the night.

The hospital routines which begin early in the morning and visiting hours do produce noise and interference with rest on the maternity floor. These problems are not solved by separating the baby from the mother. The mother needs to be allowed by hospital personnel to meet the normal needs of her healthy baby. She gains feelings of competence by taking care of her baby. She rests better when she knows that her baby has been fed and is sleeping. The mother-child relationship begins in the hospital. Even if her baby is premature there is no reason why she cannot touch him and share in his care.

It is a myth for anyone, doctor or parent, to assume that each baby in the nursery is actually watched constantly, that his needs for holding and feeding are met in the nursery, and that his care is a medical responsibility which no ordinary mortal could assume. The care system has not been set up that way to provide individual care continually. The use of monitoring equipment would not be the answer for providing constant observation either, but would simply offer another way of dehumanizing the care of the new baby. Only recently have some nurseries begun to be less routinized with less emphasis on housekeeping chores. If they are breast-fed, babies are more likely to be brought to their mothers when they need to be brought.

After the baby is born there is an emotional adjustment to be made along with the physical changes which occur after birth. The woman realizes that she is both wife and mother. The man is now a father. She needs affection from him and he needs affection and appreciation from her. The woman feels more dependent than usual during the pregnancy, labor, and delivery, and also after the birth. If she feels neglected she finds it harder to meet the needs of her husband and baby. The baby does not really require a relationship with both of his parents immediately, but the father's feelings and attitudes matter very much. Especially at this time parents should share their feelings with each other, not just take a trip down the hall to peer at the baby through the glass of the nursery window. Family-centered maternity care offers valuable opportunities for the new parents. The father can touch and hold his baby. When the time comes to go home he should be the person to take his wife and baby home from the hospital.

The mother may have some feelings of depression at some time during the early days or weeks. The prepared childbirth experience with the emotional support which it provides is a great help in preventing or reducing these feelings which are so common in the traditional childbirth experience. There are physical adjustments and factors not entirely known which have been offered as reasons for the traditional depression feelings after childbirth. The dependence of the new baby on her reminds the mother, even if her memories are not entirely conscious, of her own childhood when she was totally dependent on maternal care. Her needs may not have been adequately met by her parents. The ability to establish a satisfying relationship with her baby following a satisfying childbirth experience, instead of trying to withdraw from parenthood, can be a help for feelings of depression.

Parents usually want to plan for someone to help in the home after mother and baby come home from the hospital. They should make sure that this person is someone with whom the mother feels comfortable and someone who will not intrude on the parent-child relationship or the husband-wife relationship. Otherwise, the mother will feel inadequate, lonely, and worried about the unknown responsibilities of parenthood. The help is to enable the mother or father to be with the baby. Its purpose is not that of the care of the baby. Sometimes new fathers do some of the essential household tasks in the early days in addition to joining their wives in the care of the new child. Many couples now prefer to share the care of the new baby as equally as possible.

Nursing the baby usually gives the mother a psychological boost after the excitement of birth is over, especially if she is helped with any problems which may occur in the early days. If she is not helped she can feel discouraged and inadequate.

Within hours after birth the physical discomforts of the postpartum period may begin. Women are often surprised. Their fears have centered around labor and delivery and they have not known very much about what happens after delivery. After a while the episiotomy stitches begin to hurt. Somewhere around the same time some women will find that they have difficulty in emptying the bladder, especially if they have had spinal anesthesia. Those who have voided during labor and delivered spontaneously may not have this problem. If it occurs the woman can alternately tighten and relax her perineum and then "let everything go" as she releases the muscles of her perineum.

Women often complain of constipation after delivery. Since an enema has usually been given upon admission to the hospital there is no need to worry about that until the third day.

Very soon after the baby is born women are introduced to "peri care." "Peri care" is the care of the perineum after the baby is born. Hospital practices vary concerning the care of the perineum. Cotton balls and water may be used for cleaning. Sitz baths help to take away the soreness from the stitches.

Cramps during the first few days after delivery are more likely to be noticed after a second or subsequent baby than they are with a first baby, probably because the muscle tone of the uterus is not as good after the uterus has once been stretched. They can be very painful, but they seldom occur after the third or fourth day following birth. Shots of an oxytocic substance given after delivery to contract the uterus increase the severity of the cramps. Nursing the baby also causes cramps at first. Shots may not be needed if the woman is nursing frequently from birth and may even be undesirable if she is producing her own oxytocin. During those first days the mother can find herself trying to hold and feed a baby with sore stitches, cramps, and maybe sore nipples and engorged breasts too.

Most of the involution, or shrinking, of the uterus occurs during the first two weeks. After delivery it weighs two pounds. At the end of a week it weighs one pound. By five or six weeks, amazingly, it has returned to the size and weight of a pear. Its remarkable growth is caused by the increased size of the muscle fibers, not by an increased number of fibers. Its return to normal size takes longer for bottle-feeding than for breast-feeding women.

Breast pain or discomfort at first is common whether or not women nurse their babies. Changes in the breasts begin to be noticed a couple of days after birth. Support for the breasts will help to promote comfort and there is also the need to prevent or relieve engorgement of the breasts as described in Chapter VI.

As the lining of the uterus is shrugged off after delivery, there is a discharge from the uterus called the lochia. At first it is reddish, then brownish. It lasts two to four weeks, the length of time being shortened if the mother is breast-feeding her baby. The amount of the discharge gradually diminishes. Douching is not necessary nor is it recommended unless ordered by the doctor.

Obstetricians often recommend exercises to their patients after the baby is born. Some exercises should be started in the hospital, but the word "exercise" should not conjure up some form of gymnastics. Care must be taken to avoid putting too much stress on muscles too soon. The exercises done in the hospital help the circulation and help the uterus to return to good position.

The pelvic floor exercise and the pelvic rock which were practiced prenatally come back into use again. The pelvic floor exercise is needed to tighten up the perineal muscles. This exercise also speeds the healing of the episiotomy by increasing circulation to that part of the body. It can be started soon after birth.

After a day or two she might do the pelvic rock while lying on her back. Women often like this exercise. Deep breathing is done and as the breath is drawn in the back is arched slightly. As the breath is slowly exhaled, the woman pulls inward and upward on her lower abdominal muscles while flattening her lower back against the bed.

After delivery if the woman lies on her abdomen with a pillow under her hips, the uterus is helped to return to good position. Another exercise can also be done immediately after birth. She can lie on her back in bed and bend and stretch her ankles, rolling the feet in a circular motion in both directions. This exercise is for the circulation.

The day after delivery the mother can slowly tighten her abdominal muscles while lying on her back and raise her head from the pillow occasionally, taking care not to place any sudden pull on the abdominal muscles. Sometimes the mother tightens her abdominal muscles and holds the tension for a few seconds before releasing them without raising her head from the pillow.

After a few days, or perhaps a week, an exercise for the waistline can be started. The woman lies on her back and draws up one knee. She then twists the knee over to reach the bed on the opposite side. If the exercise is started at home it is better to do it on the floor. After practicing with one knee, both knees can be drawn up and twisted toward the floor.

Like the exercises for pregnancy and birth, the ones childbirth educators suggest are not difficult or unpleasant exercises which are a chore to do. They are effective without being strenuous. Childbirth classes often teach perhaps two or three exercises to do after the baby is born. Ebner,[2] an English physical therapist, has a section on postpartum restoration in her book. The Maternity Center Association[3] also published a booklet which has information on exercises to be done after childbirth.

An exercise, often called the lactation exercise, is used to increase the circulation to the chest area and breasts. It feels good to do, and it may aid milk production as it increases the blood supply to the chest area. The arms are bent and the fists are on the shoulders. Elbows are close to the sides. The elbows are then brought forward toward each other pressing against the sides of the breasts, up and around to make a circle. The woman usually does this exercise while sitting cross-legged.

Leg-raising exercises in which the legs are kept straight and lifted off the floor should not be done during the early weeks after birth. They could cause damage to the abdominal muscles by exerting too much pull on them. There are other abdominal exercises which are preferable and adequate for regaining abdominal tone such as the ones just described.

Heavy lifting should not be done during the early weeks either. When lifting is done the back should be straight, not bent. Work surfaces should not be so low that they cause back strain.

During all the postpartum period good posture is one of

the best ways of avoiding fatigue and regaining a good figure.

Intercourse after Childbirth

After the baby has been born parents will wonder about the resumption of intercourse and question the method of contraception to be used. Obstetricians give advice on intercourse during pregnancy and after delivery. There are variations in the advice given in different parts of the world, depending mostly on cultural customs and taboos. Masters and Johnson have shed some light on the subject by providing facts which were formerly unavailable. American obstetricians have prohibited intercourse for six to eight weeks before delivery and until after the six-week checkup following the delivery. There is a trend toward more flexibility in the advice given, depending on how the woman feels and on the speed of recovery after birth.

Intercourse becomes more difficult to accomplish as pregnancy advances, but it is not associated with miscarriage or harm to the baby as many couples have quite naturally feared. If the woman has a history of miscarriage, the obstetrician may take the precaution of prohibiting intercourse during the first three months of pregnancy on the days when the menstrual periods would have occurred had the woman not become pregnant. Intercourse does not initiate labor, even if it causes uterine contractions, unless the woman was ready to go into labor anyway.

After delivery, when intercourse is first attempted the couple should not be surprised if at first there are the problems of tightness and dryness of the vagina. The tightness results from the episiotomy, and if this is a real problem the obstetrician should be called. The dryness results from the fact that the normal lubrication from Bartholin's glands near the entrance of the vagina may be absent for some time after childbirth. Vaseline or contraceptive cream is used for lubrication if needed.

Ovulation is delayed by breast feeding, even though breast feeding has been found to be associated with a more rapid return of sexual interests, but breast feeding is not at all a sure method of contraception. The use of birth control pills will decrease the milk supply. The intrauterine device may cause increased bleeding after childbirth and its use will require the opinion of the obstetrician. The diaphragm is the contraceptive method used most often after childbirth. If a diaphragm has been used before pregnancy, the size should be checked by the obstetrician because a larger size may be needed after childbirth.

VI

BREAST FEEDING

Many women in the United States have never seen a baby at the breast. Women who have not had preparation for childbirth have often had mixed feelings about nursing their babies. Nursing a baby is a close physical act with deep emotional significance. Many women have not been comfortable with the idea even though they may be aware that they and their babies are missing a basic life experience. Yet seldom does it occur that a woman who has experienced prepared childbirth goes on to feed her baby with a bottle.

It might seem that breast feeding would not have to be taught, that the woman need only offer her breast to her hungry baby. This is essentially true, yet many women say that they would like to have nursed their babies but "couldn't." Sometimes they feel that their milk is inadequate in some way or that they are not "doing it right." And they may not realize that the size of the breast is of little importance in the amount of milk produced.

The appearance and contour of the breast are seen as important in our culture. Appearance is undeniably important, but after childbirth the breast also becomes a functioning, secreting organ. This situation is a new one to women and to men.

Professional curricula have taught infant formulas and bottle feeding to such an extent that many professionals have been left uncertain about counseling nursing mothers although they, of course, feel that breast feeding is desirable and the ideal way to feed a baby.

Breast feeding is often taught in childbirth education classes. Couples may find difficulty in anticipating the experience of infant feeding whether it be by breast or bottle. The baby is not yet born and the breasts are not yet secreting milk. The immediate experience for couples is birth, but women are asked very soon after birth for a decision on how they plan to feed their babies. The obstetrician may ask women during pregnancy whether they are planning to breast-feed.

Pregnancy is a time of emotional fluidity with unusual opportunities for greater self-awareness and emotional growth. The woman should feel free to change her mind at any time on the subject of infant feeding, just as she should be free to change her mind on the subject of medication during labor instead of having to choose natural childbirth or the traditional kind of medicated labor when she is still in the beginning of her pregnancy. Knowledge about breast feeding given ahead of time allows parents an opportunity to make an informed choice instead of feeling that they are being rushed into a choice which they really don't know very much about. Husbands and wives can sort out their feelings and talk about them. Besides, any difficulties women may have will most likely come during the early days or first weeks because of such situations as discouragement by other people around the new mother and lack of understanding of the baby's growth spurts and of the changes in size of the breasts as the early engorgement subsides.

In childbirth classes a mother from the previous class series often comes back to tell expectant parents what it is like to be a breast-feeding mother. The new father may come, too, to give his feelings on what it is like to be a father and how a breast-feeding baby fits into the life of the new family.

Whether or not a woman wishes to breast-feed depends partly on her husband's feelings. Before the husband can support his wife's wish to nurse, he needs to get his own questions answered. He comes to the session on breast feeding. If he sees this process as unnecessary or is disturbed by it, or if he feels that the baby is depriving him of attention from his wife, then an element of disharmony is immediately introduced.

If his child is to be nursed, the new father helps to provide a home atmosphere which will protect his wife from unnecessary interruptions and interferences. He helps his wife feel confident in caring for the new baby instead of surrendering her mothering role to work in the kitchen, for example, while the helping person in the home sits comfortably in the living room rocking the baby. Prepared husbands encourage their wives to take care of themselves by eating high-quality food and by resting when the baby is sleeping. They also help wives decide which household chores are non-essential during the early days and weeks.

Early feeding experiences are important to mother and

baby. The mother's ego cannot help but be involved. If her baby will not suck, or if he continues to cry, she needs to know why and what she can do. As parents learn what to do they get satisfaction from watching a new little person become satisfied and grow on the milk produced by his mother.

Just as childbirth is a skill to be learned, breast feeding is also a skill to be learned. It is not just a technical or a physiological process; it involves also the establishment of a relationship between two people, the mother and the baby. Feeding the baby is not entirely a chore for the mother. The nursing mother wants her full breasts to be emptied by the baby. The woman's confidence in her ability to breast-feed is vital in achieving a feeding relationship which is satisfying to mother and baby. Too often when doubts and problems have appeared, the advice given by relatives, pediatrician, nurse, or obstetrician has been to switch to a bottle.

Hospital routines traditionally have been a handicap in establishing breast feeding. The baby's long hours in the central nursery are not conducive to bringing in an early milk supply. Separation from the new baby also affects the mother's desire to nurse. The hospital feedings have been spaced almost as far apart as are adult meals and they have usually met neither the baby's nor the mother's needs. Family-centered care now provides a solution to this problem because it allows more access to the baby than was formerly possible. The increased flexibility in feeding babies according to their needs has brought an added bonus to the hospital maternity floor. It is quieter and more restful.

The method of breast feeding taught in classes and described in the following pages has been used by hospitals and has been sought out by mothers who thought that they could not nurse a baby. The teaching is based largely on the knowledge and experience of the La Leche League.[1] This organization was formed in 1957 by a group of mothers with the support of a medical advisory board for the purpose of helping women to breast-feed. A manual[2] was prepared and has been widely distributed. At present over a thousand local La Leche groups, most of them in the United States, are offering counseling service to women. The approach offered is a flexible and relaxed one. It is not really new, but it offers help in overcoming the traditional obstacles which have caused many people to consider breast feeding a time-consuming task which is hard to do and which can be accomplished only by certain women. Newton[3] and Haire[4] are among those who have published material on breast feeding based on this new approach.

The new mother may get conflicting advice about breast feeding after her baby is born just as she will about many aspects of mothering and parenthood. Some obstetricians and pediatricians do have some doubts about the advice given by childbirth education associations and the La Leche groups. They do not believe that virtually all women can nurse a baby. They do not agree that there is no need for soap or antiseptic substances on the nipples. They feel that women should not nurse during a breast infection. They also feel that solid food should be introduced with less delay. Other physicians stand behind the method of breast feeding which is being taught to mothers. These physicians have seen flat-chested women blossom forth to produce an abundance of milk. They feel that soap on nipples contributes to soreness and drying of sensitive tissue, and they feel that if there should be an infection within the breast, then the milk should be kept flowing. The baby is not harmed by a breast infection in the mother.

The glib remark that bottle feeding is as good as breast feeding is not entirely true, although bottle babies will be satisfied and will thrive. There are advantages to breast feeding and the advantages are not all for the baby. The mother recovers faster from childbirth because nursing encourages the production of oxytocin, the hormone which acts to help the uterus return to its normal size.

The need for resuscitation measures is unlikely with the unmedicated baby. The suction bulb often inserted into his mouth after delivery may not be needed either. There is little need for concern about a baby who sucks and swallows, even if he only sucks for a minute or less. The colostrum present in the breasts at birth offers both protein and protection from infection and, because early sucking encourages the milk to come in early, the baby's weight loss during the first few days is minimized.

There are other little-known benefits of breast feeding, all of them documented in the Haire manual.[5] Breast milk is a protection against infant illness and infant mortality. Its lower solute load puts less of a burden on the baby's immature kidneys. It increases his chances of avoiding all manner of health hazards such as upper respiratory infections, gastrointestinal infections, hay fever, eczema, and asthma. It is a protection against dental caries later in life. Its most dramatic benefits are its protection against allergy.

Cow's milk is one of the most allergy-producing foods there is for babies who have any tendency toward allergic reactions. Allergy to breast milk has never been satisfactorily demonstrated.[6] So-called allergy to human milk is found to be due to substances transmitted through the milk, not to the milk protein itself. Even if there should be an Rh problem there is no reason not to nurse the baby. Rarely, a food or other substance such as food additives eaten by the mother may disagree with the baby. The baby may react to vitamin solutions given to him or to his mother. Fluoride solutions have been known to cause a reaction. Occasionally a baby's early difficulty has been misdiagnosed as an allergy.

DDT does get into the mother's milk. Children today are exposed to DDT from the beginning of their lives. Protection from DDT can come only from essential environmental controls. One thing a woman can do for herself is to eat less animal fat because DDT is stored in the fat of animals.

Since human milk is a more complete food than diluted cow's milk and carbohydrate formulas, solid foods are not required as early as they are with bottle babies. After a while iron and vitamins C and D will have to come from other sources, but many pediatricians feel that solid foods are not required until the baby is over three months old. Solid foods are not well assimilated by the very young baby. They may produce allergic reactions and they also interfere with the sucking response which is essential for an abundant milk supply. The Committee on Nutrition of the American Academy of Pediatrics makes the statement, "No nutritional advantage or disadvantage has yet been proven for supplementing adequate milk diets with solid foods in the first three or four months of life."[7] This statement has not been revised since it was made in 1958. There is another reason for not urging solid foods earlier than necessary. Baby foods, too, are now made from fruits and vegetables which have been heavily sprayed with the hard pesticides which accumulate in the body instead of breaking down as one would expect poisonous substances to do.

Human milk as it is secreted is sterile but requires refrigeration if it is to be stored. It can also be frozen. Human milk normally looks thinner than cow's milk and is bluish in color. It tastes sweeter than cow's milk. As it digests in the baby's stomach the curds formed are soft and small, and there is less residue after digestion than there is with cow's milk. Because less air is swallowed while feeding there is less need for burping the baby.

Many pregnant women express a fear of being "tied down." The new mother will be "tied down" for a few weeks anyway after the birth regardless of how she feeds the baby. Babies do need their parents' time and attention, but they also need to rest and sleep. Breast feeding requires that the woman eat nutritious foods, have a chance to rest and to be relieved of unnecessary obligations. These are needs of hers which she might not otherwise feel entitled to meet. Her physical closeness with her baby is only temporary. Gradually the baby becomes less needful of physical contact and feeding as the weeks and months pass by. He moves toward more independence and wishes for social contacts.

Care of the Breasts

Breast feeding does not harm the female figure and may even improve it. However, because the breasts are enlarged, especially soon after birth, a supportive bra should be worn for comfort, especially if the woman is concerned about possible sagging of the breasts. There should be no constriction of breast tissue either. The supportive bra should be worn during pregnancy and after birth. It may be worn at night as well as during the day during the first days after delivery. The process of aging or overweight can cause sagging, but it is not due to breast feeding if ordinary care is taken.

During pregnancy the nipples should be washed gently with a rough washcloth, taking care to avoid irritation. The nipples can be pulled out and twisted gently, especially if they are flat or inverted as they are on some women.

A shower and clean clothes each day provide adequate cleanliness for the nursing mother. There is no need for any other cleansing of the breast. No soap, alcohol, or tincture of benzoin should be used on the nipples because these substances take the fat out of the skin and invite soreness of the nipples. Lanolin can be used on the nipples and need not be washed off before feeding the baby. The hands do require thorough washing before feedings because they can carry harmful bacteria.

After feedings the nipples should be air-dried if possible. Sometimes the mother leaves the bra flaps of the nursing bra down under a loose blouse to allow circulation of air. Plastic shields in the bra should never be used because these will encourage softening and soreness of the nipples and will also encourage the growth of bacteria. The leaking of milk for which the shields were designed can be stopped in other ways. The leaking will stop by itself after the first few weeks.

"How to Do It"

At first both mother and baby are uncertain as to how to get started. If the baby's cheek is stroked or placed against the breast, he will turn toward the source of stimulation, but if the nipple is pushed into his mouth he will probably resist. The mother makes sure that the breast is not pressing his nose to block his breathing. Sometimes this causes babies to struggle and pull away without the new mother realizing why. She presses the breast tissue away from his nose with her finger.

If the mother receives medication to dry up her milk after delivery and then changes her mind about nursing, she can overcome the effects of this medication by frequent nursing. If the mother has received a substantial dose of medication during labor, the baby may be slower in learning to nurse.

The baby is encouraged to take as much of the areola around the nipple as possible. His jaws will then come down where they should on the milk-collecting sinuses behind the nipple. Also, if he takes in the area around the nipple there will be less nipple soreness.

During nursing the baby may be supported on his mother's lap on top of a pillow. If the mother wishes, especially at first when the stitch area is still sore, she may lie on her side with her lower arm around her baby's head. Later, at home, she may also enjoy this position as she feeds the baby in bed. She can cuddle him, talk to him, and at times doze or watch television.

During pregnancy parents learn about the anatomy and physiology of the breast. The milk is secreted deep within the breast in the alveoli. These alveoli look like bunches of grapes and are located near the chest wall. The milk passes down to the collecting sinuses behind the nipple. About 15 to 20 ducts open onto the surface of the nipple. The contour of the breast depends mostly on the distribution of fat and is not determined by the milk-producing glands.

As the baby is put to breast he does not suck as he does on the bottle. Actually, he thrusts his tongue forward to draw the nipple in. His jaws then compress the area around the nipple, causing the milk to be squeezed out through the nipple ducts.

As he nurses, a neurohormonal reflex called the let-down reflex encourages the pituitary gland to secrete oxytocin into the blood stream where it acts on the tiny milk sacs, causing them to tighten. The milk is squeezed down to the sinuses behind the nipple where the baby can get it. Oxytocin is an important human hormone. It is involved in male ejaculation, female orgasm,[8] labor, delivery, the shrinking of the uterus after delivery and, finally, it triggers the let-down reflex.

The let-down reflex during nursing is essential to breast feeding. It may be initiated by the sight of the new baby or by the sound of his cry as well as by sucking. As the milk is about to let down the mother feels a tingling sensation. The milk may actually spurt out of the nipple. The reflex requires about thirty to ninety seconds. It is inhibited by embarrassment, disturbance, or distraction of the mother. Therefore, especially in the beginning, she needs privacy to nurse and a feeling of confidence in order to let down her milk.

At each feeding the baby is offered both breasts to give each breast the stimulation it needs to produce milk and to give the baby enough milk. Some women are still told to nurse on only one side at a feeding. This practice encourages engorgement in the unused breast and contributes to a diminished milk supply. Most women must nurse on both breasts at each feeding. At each feeding the starting side is alternated. If the baby was started on the left side for one feeding, he will be offered the right breast first at the next feeding. The woman can often tell which breast needs to be emptied first. To switch sides the mother breaks the suction by pressing her finger against the corner of the breast to let in air. The nipple can then come out easily without pulling it away from the baby.

The breast is empty when the baby sucks without swallowing regularly. At first he may swallow with every suck. Soon he swallows with every other suck or every few sucks. He sucks even when there is no milk, oftentimes, just to satisfy the need to suck. The breast is never completely empty, however, or does not remain so, because milk is continuously secreted. The more the baby sucks the more milk is secreted.

At first the baby's time on the breast is limited to help avoid nipple soreness. The baby must therefore be fed more often. There is some controversy over the amount of correlation between length of sucking time and soreness. Some soreness may be unavoidable. The baby is usually nursed frequently, but not for long stretches of time. He is given less than five minutes on a side, perhaps only three minutes, to start. Later he will spend ten minutes or longer on a side. The baby gets most of the milk fairly promptly so he is not short-changed very much on the amount of milk he gets at each feeding. The breast does get fairly well emptied, a factor which is very important in building up the milk supply. After the first few days the baby is allowed plenty of time to suck. The time limitation at first is not an interfering factor in building up milk production because the supply is more dependent on the frequency of letting down milk than on long periods of sucking.

Breast babies swallow less air than bottle babies, but at some time during the feeding, after the major portion of the baby's hunger has been satisfied, he should be held with his stomach against his mother's shoulder. His back is then patted and rubbed to get up any air bubbles in his stomach. A bubble may make him think that his stomach is full when it is not, and it can also cause him discomfort and some regurgitation of milk. Sometimes some milk may come up with the bubble. He can also be burped by sitting in his mother's lap. She puts one hand on his stomach as he sits across her lap and rubs his back with the other hand. As the baby leans forward over his mother's hand, he must be able to support his own head. His mother may be able to help support his head if she leans slightly backward to allow him to rest the side of his head against her body. At the end of the feeding the baby is again burped.

Engorgement of the breast is less likely to occur if the baby is nursed promptly and frequently from the time of birth instead of being kept in the nursery and fed at infrequent intervals. Some women, though, do seem to get engorged more easily than others. The same woman may notice it more with one baby than with another. Engorgement is not directly related to the milk supply. When the engorgement is relieved and the breast again becomes smaller, the milk has not gone. The engorgement results from hormonal changes and an increased blood supply to the breasts a couple of days after birth as the milk starts to come in. The breast becomes hard and the baby cannot grasp it because the nipple is pulled taut. If he tries the woman will feel severe pain, and the baby may cry in frustration. The mother resolves this situation by massaging the breast from the armpit toward the nipple, doing this on all sides of both breasts. She then places her fingers at either side of the areola and compresses the sinuses behind the nipple. The nipple is then drawn forward in a milking motion. As the mother feels the milk letting down and the breast softening she puts the baby to breast.

During the early weeks of nursing many women find that milk leaks from their breasts. The amount of leaking is no indicator of the milk supply. When the leaking stops, as it usually does after the first weeks, the milk supply has not decreased. Women may have leaking with one baby and not have leaking with another baby. It can be controlled by pressure with the hand or forearm on the nipple. If the baby is nursing on one breast and there is leaking from the other, the application of pressure will control it. A man's handkerchief placed in the bra to absorb the moisture works out well and also allows air to reach the nipple.

Frequency of Feeding

The supply of milk is closely related to the frequency of feeding. If the baby is fed on a need-satisfaction basis the supply will adapt to his needs. If there is a growth spurt and the baby becomes fussy, he will nurse more often. The milk supply then builds up to meet the increased need and the baby goes back to more infrequent feedings again.

If he is teething and takes less milk temporarily, the supply will build up rapidly again when he needs it.

The feeding pattern is variable and differs very much from one baby to another and in the same baby as he grows. It is not possible to schedule feedings, especially at first, and it is a hardship on mother and baby to try. The feeding need of the newborn is very urgent. He awakes, grimaces in apparent pain, and cries. The hunger contractions build up suddenly instead of gradually as in the older baby and adult. Later the baby will develop more of a schedule and the mother can help him adapt to the needs of the family, at least to an extent.

The milk comes in from two to four days after delivery when the hormone prolactin begins circulating in the blood, but if the mother nurses frequently from the beginning the milk may come in sooner than two days. It may come in within twenty-four hours. It builds up from a few ounces each day to more than a quart per day in a few weeks. Mothers have found that they can nurse twins, so closely related is the supply to the demand, but if the mother does nurse twins she will find that she is unusually hungry and thirsty and will require an extra meal each day. She will probably take a drink of milk or juice as she sits down to nurse.

The first day home from the hospital the mother often has less milk than she had, perhaps, the day before. When the milk supply is not yet really established and is just barely coming in well, it is more easily diminished by changes or an unusual amount of activity. At about six weeks there is a growth spurt and the mother may wonder for a brief time whether she has enough milk. At about three months is another time when the baby may be fussy.

At that time, too, he is starting to develop more of an interest in the world around him. When the baby needs to be fed more often than usual, the mother simply washes her hands, picks up the baby, and nurses him. If she wears a blouse or sweater she can pull it up from the bottom and nurse fairly unobtrusively with the baby covering her midriff. If she has a baby carrier made in the form of a sling she does not even have to sit down to nurse him, although she usually relaxes and gives the baby her attention during feeding time.

At some time early in life the baby may need to be fed every hour for a few feedings, but this is only temporary and should not discourage the new mother. The ill baby may need to be fed more frequently because he may take less milk at each feeding and because he also needs comfort. If his nose is stuffy it is harder for him to nurse.

Babies are generally fed every two or three hours in the beginning. Breast-fed babies are fed more frequently than bottle babies because breast milk is more digestible than formula and does not stay in the stomach as long. Breast milk also contains less fat.

It may seem almost too obvious to say that the food the mother eats is important to the milk supply and to her feeling of well-being, yet many women come home from the hospital without realizing that their fatigue and difficulty in satisfying the baby are related to the food they are eating. Many people do not realize how much protein is required by the pregnant woman and the nursing mother. A woman who is nursing a baby should have in the neighborhood of 100 grams of protein each day. For purposes of illustration, a 3-ounce serving of cooked lean beef will give her only 19 grams of protein. She needs more meat, and also plenty of milk and cottage cheese. She also needs vitamins. Many women find that an easy way of adding B vitamins to the diet is to use wheat germ and nutritional yeast such as brewer's yeast (not the baking yeast found in grocery stores). These foods definitely lack taste appeal and must be mixed with other foods, but they often seem to result in a dramatically increased milk supply. They do contain some protein also. The woman who nurses needs a plentiful supply of eggs, fruits (especially citrus fruits), and vegetables. She should try to avoid the so-called "junk foods" which are high in carbohydrates because the consumption of carbohydrates in these foods is associated with a diminished supply of B vitamins and is also associated with a diminished milk supply. Breast milk contains a generous amount of vitamin E. Because vitamin E is almost totally lacking in most American diets (one source is wheat germ oil), women are beginning to add a vitamin E supplement to their diets.

Other factors besides inadequate food or inadequate sucking by the baby can interfere with the milk supply. After emotional stress or too much activity by the mother the baby will need to be fed more often for a while to build up the milk supply again. Also, solid foods given to the baby too soon may diminish the milk supply, especially if given during the first three months. It is better, too, not to supplement breast milk with formula for an evening away from the baby until the breast milk is well established. Any liquids given to the baby besides milk are often given by eye dropper as he is held to the breast. This prevents interference with sucking at the breast. Babies can learn very easily to prefer the bottle because the food comes to them more easily with less need to use their facial muscles.

The supply of milk is also diminished by the use of

birth control pills, antihistamines, or diuretics. No medicines should be taken while nursing a baby without discussing the situation with the doctor.

The baby's hunger varies from feeding to feeding. If there is a question about whether or not he is getting enough milk, the general rule seems to be that he is adequately supplied if (1) he has at least six wet diapers per day with pale, not concentrated, urine, assuming that he is not being given water and (2) he goes three to four hours between feedings after the early weeks when breast feeding is becoming established.

Occasionally parents are unlucky enough to have a colicky baby even if the baby is breast-fed, a situation exhausting for parents and painful for the baby. The causes are not entirely clear. Colic may be due to small, immature digestive organs and it can be made worse if the atmosphere around the baby is tense. The breast-feeding mother does have an advantage over the bottle-feeding mother. The baby can be given frequent, smaller feedings. He can be held and allowed to suck on the breast with less chance of overfeeding than if he is receiving a bottle of formula. He cries often and needs to suck but does not always need milk each time he cries. When he does not need milk, at least not in large amounts, he can be offered the emptier breast. Colic is usually gone by the time the baby is three months old.

Coping with Problems

When problems are described they can make breast feeding appear to be full of pitfalls instead of an easy and satisfying way of feeding a baby, but parents need to be prepared for possible problems. When information is needed, it is needed immediately, not tomorrow or next week. Most problems come in the early days when breast feeding is becoming established and they can be prevented or alleviated by knowing what to do. Even if a woman does not entirely succeed in avoiding pain and problems, the difficulties can be expected to last only a matter of days.

Breast inflammations or infections can occur after delivery even if the mother is not nursing. If she is nursing she should not stop because this may make the infection worse. The mother will nurse less frequently on that breast, but she will keep the milk flowing. She should rest and she should also ask her doctor about applying heat or taking an antibiotic to halt the infection and bring her temperature back down. She must step up her fluid intake, too.

Occasionally a clogged milk duct may be confused with an infection. It feels like a lump and can be relieved by massage. Its cause may be a tight bra.

Soreness is the most common problem, not infections. The woman who is nursing a baby should take preventive measures even if soreness has not yet developed. The skin is tender because in daily life it is not exposed to air and weather. The nipples are washed with water to help make sure that all the ducts in the nipple are open, not caked with milk. The baby is nursed as soon and as frequently as the hospital permits and the baby demands. The baby sucks often, but not long at a time at first. The nipples are air-dried, especially at first, whether or not any soreness has developed. Lanolin may be used on the nipples.

If something more than these usual procedures are required, there are other practical helps to try. Exposure of the breast to a 25-watt bulb may help to heal a sore or cracked nipple. Hair dryers have been used successfully, too. Sun on the bared breast through an open window is a great help.

Soreness in the early days may require that the baby be nursed less frequently on the side with the most soreness, especially if the soreness has been allowed to develop into a crack in the nipple. The milk does need to be kept flowing. It can be expressed out by hand or started by hand with a manual milking motion before the baby is put onto the breast. Sometimes the baby can be put onto the breast at a slightly different angle, but still making sure that he takes in not only the nipple but also the areola around the nipple.

The uncertainties of the early days have often discouraged unprepared women unnecessarily from carrying out their initial wish to nurse their babies which they expressed after delivery. Other women have not even dared to express the wish to try breast feeding, so certain are they that it would be too difficult or that they would face some form of disapproval. Some hospital staff people have the special knowledge required to help mothers. Childbirth education associations often have nursing mothers groups as part of their program in addition to teaching breast feeding in the classes which they sponsor. These and the local La Leche groups make themselves available on a round-the-clock basis to parents who seldom have access to relatives possessing the knowledge and skill associated with breast feeding.

VII

The Childbirth Education Class

Unlike the earlier natural childbirth classes, the childbirth education classes now are couple-oriented although women may come alone. As a reflection of the changing times, in some parts of the country not all of the couples are married, but they do seek a shared experience.

Although classes are important to get the full benefit of the experience, nurses and labor coaches do find that they can help couples who have not attended a class and even couples who have never heard of childbirth education. Nurses and labor coaches offer human presence, companionship, and information. They also offer help with relaxation, positioning, and controlled breathing. When this kind of help is given, the usual dose of medication is frequently not needed even if couples did not attend a class.

The Instructor's Dilemma

The childbirth education instructor often finds herself in a dilemma which requires some skill to resolve. Shall she "tell it like it is" or will parent confidence in hospital care be shaken when couples find out that their expectations cannot always be fulfilled and are even seen as idealistic or impossible? Couples who have already had a baby will be aware of the instructor's dilemma almost immediately as they embark on a series of classes in areas where family-centered care, which is really patient-centered care, is not readily available.

It is desirable for women to be able to enter the hospital relaxed and confident of what to expect, feeling that their needs will be met as far as possible. Yet often a surgical patient entering the hospital can know more about what to expect than can the maternity patient. For example, the husband may have been told that he could stay with his wife but finds that the labor area designated for prepared couples is filled and therefore he cannot stay. Or he may leave during the routine shave and enema which is still usually required upon admission or he may leave while his wife is being examined during labor, and the nurse may forget to call him back because she was busy, forgot, or was not aware that he was planning to stay. Although nurses who have observed childbirth classes and who have had experience with conscious, participating childbirth may know what to say and do for women in labor, the situation can occur in which the woman does not receive emotional support during labor and may feel very much alone. She may not be told of her progress, how far dilated she is, or reassured that she is doing well with her techniques. She may not be offered pillows for proper positioning during labor and delivery. Ice chips may not be available, and the couple may have to use wet paper towels or lollipops which they have brought from home if the wife's mouth feels dry as she uses the breathing techniques.

In some hospitals expectant couples may want to know ahead of time about the possibility of the use of fetal monitoring equipment which makes a continuous recording of the contractions and the baby's heartbeat. The equipment is more accurate than the stethoscope. Doctors can even sit in the doctors' lounge and watch the recording from there. There is more than one kind of equipment. It may be something attached to the abdomen or it may be the kind which is inserted into the vagina. Even the kind that simply magnifies the sound of the baby's heartbeat so that it can be heard across the room can be an unsettling experience. Parents sometimes assume mistakenly that the use of this equipment indicates a problem with their baby.

As yet there is no evidence that it adds safety and is the change needed to improve the infant death rate. It does have its uses. In case of a sudden need for a Caesarean section it serves a purpose. For the high-risk patient it may indeed increase safety. But in some ways its use can be compared to the theoretical situation of the overprotective parent who locks his school-aged child in the yard because he might get run over by street traffic. Yes, he might. The question is, should all women be subjected to this?

Monitoring equipment has provided some useful information about labor contractions and their effects on the fetal heart rate. When labor is being stimulated excessively by pitocin or other oxytocic substance, the infant's distress will be shown on the monitor. Then, when this is observed, the stimulation of labor is discontinued as recommended in the literature on monitoring,[1] and the woman turned onto her side to improve her circulation. If conduction anesthesia lowers the mother's blood pressure, the results can also be seen on the monitor.

The electrodes are introduced into the vagina, one under the baby's scalp and one on the uterus. There may be some discomfort from this procedure. A strap is placed around the mother's leg to hold the leg plate, which is connected to the monitor. The baby will have two pinpricks on his scalp after delivery. These will heal in a couple of days.

The woman can move and change to the side position, but she does feel hampered by the equipment and she cannot help but be afraid of dislodging it. The real problem is that she feels helpless and finds it harder to relax. She feels immobilized.

The woman in labor may also be given fluids intravenously even though this procedure is not usually needed for healthy women who are not ill or dehydrated. It prevents women from moving freely and, of course, also prevents them from getting up to go to the bathroom.

The woman can be in the position of having monitoring equipment in her vagina, an intravenous needle in her arm, and an epidural anesthesia catheter in her back! The *American Journal of Nursing* says, "The nurse working in labor and delivery today finds herself in the center of technological marvels which may overwhelm her patients."[2] This is indeed true. The procedures involved are not simple nor is the equipment. There is the danger, however, of inducing those young couples already turned off by the idea of having a baby in the hospital to have their babies at home. They should know that they do have the right to refuse these procedures if they wish.

During labor the woman may get an excessive dose of medication instead of the light dose she may require to take the edge off the sharpness of the contractions. If she shows indecision during the difficult period of transition, she may get spinal or other anesthesia which she does not really want or require instead of the coaching and comfort measures she desires.

Although the hands of conscious, prepared women are not usually strapped down in the delivery room with stout leather wristlets, sometimes this does happen. Some women are not bothered by having their hands strapped down. Others are made tense and anxious. Of course, these restraints were designed for unconscious women, but some doctors and nurses still fear that the woman might touch the sterile sheets draped over her legs even if she is told not to, or that she might touch the birth area, especially if she reaches down for the baby. It is a normal response to reach toward the baby and some obstetricians like to see a new mother respond in this way. Others are unaccustomed to this response and are bothered by it.

After the delivery it is possible that the baby may be wheeled from the delivery room before the mother and father have really had a chance to see him. The mother may not be able to see her baby again for a number of hours while he remains in his nursery crib. Women sometimes worry that something is wrong with the baby if he cannot be brought to them. If the window shades of the nursery are pulled down parents cannot even see their baby through the glass. When babies are brought out to mothers they may be dropped off like bundles of laundry with no explanations or help for new mothers because the babies are all distributed at the same time.

The new mother may or may not get help with breast feeding. Usually the nursing mother can have her baby for a night feeding, although she may have to ask for this. Her obstetrician may leave orders for her baby to be brought to her at night. On the other hand, she may be told that she needs her sleep even though her breasts are hard and tender and she needs to nurse before she can sleep. The mother may have planned for a modified rooming-in arrangement with her baby, but the rooms designated as rooming-in rooms may be filled, in which case she cannot nurse when she feels the need or when the baby cries with hunger. It is true that the possibility of infection is greater in the hospital than at home, but the antiseptic substances sometimes required by hospital procedures do encourage soreness and cracking of the nipples.

Expectant parents entering the hospital may have some or none of the above difficulties, or they may have other difficulties. If they object, they may disturb relationships among hospital personnel, who then may label the patient as uncooperative.

The differences in different hospitals are due largely to attitudes rather than more money and staff in some hospitals than others. Some aspects of the maternity experience are affected by which staff member happens to be on duty at a critical time. Women going to the same hospital and the same doctor may have different experiences, partly due to chance and partly due to their own efforts.

Problems of parents can be more difficult to solve because there is fragmentation of maternity care with no one individual totally responsible for the maternity experience as it affects the whole family. The woman's contacts with her obstetrician are often brief and he is unaware of the hour-to-hour care of mother and baby. After leaving the hospital mother and baby ordinarily have no medical contacts until the baby is six weeks old, when the mother gets a postpartum checkup and the baby has his first pediatric office visit.

Therefore it is important that parents learn how to enlist the cooperation of all who are involved in their care. Parents must communicate with the obstetrician before they choose a doctor and a hospital as well as with the obstetrician and nurses at the hospital after they arrive. Prepared childbirth is not a do-it-yourself project even if parents are educated about childbirth.

Parent needs are not unrealistic, but parents cannot assume that everything will be taken care of automatically by their obstetrician. Parents will have to do some work. Parent needs are discussed in classes, not to make couples apprehensive but to help them. Otherwise they may later feel that the class, the hospital, and the obstetrician let them down and they may be very critical of the care.

The childbirth instructor cannot guarantee that couples will have their needs met, but she can often help them solve their problems. Whether the instructor is employed by a hospital or by a community group, she can be expected to understand hospital and parent needs in a way which will help couples in class to negotiate the care system to their satisfaction and that of the hospital. Parents learn how hospital care is organized and how it governs the actions of professional workers giving the care. Parents learn who is responsible for each aspect of the care and they have the opportunity for more satisfying relationships with the obstetrician, the nurses, and the pediatrician unless the goals of parents and professionals are very different.

If there is strong resistance to parent participation by the obstetrician or in the hospital they have chosen, couples should know this ahead of time. The husband and wife make the decision to change doctors or hospitals if they feel that it is important to them. The instructor helps them to feel all right about making their decision. She reassures them that their needs are important.

There is still resistance to family-centered care even though it is fundamentally safer than conventional care and even though it offers satisfactions to parents and professionals. The resistance centers around certain concerns in addition to the natural resistance to change. The public has not yet been educated to request the new type of care in large numbers and hospitals can feel that they would be giving two types of care. Some mothers would have access to their husbands and babies if they wished and others would not. Some hospital personnel are distressed by the presence of husbands. One of the original concerns of hospitals was the fear of infection until careful thinking was done and studies showed that family-centered care was a protection against infection.

Consumers have become more knowledgeable about health care and institutional care in general. They are less tolerant of frustrations than they used to be. The issues involved in maternity care have come into public awareness more slowly, but numbers of professionals are interested in improving maternity care from the parent and baby viewpoints so that couples who invest some time and energy can usually find a dignified and gratifying childbirth experience.

The instructor fills a community health education role in addition to that of teaching parents about childbirth and helping them obtain the type of care they desire. She informs others in the community about what is taught to couples. She makes visits to hospitals and obstetricians. She talks with student nurses. She helps to bridge the gap between the hospital and the community by inviting hospital nurses, medical and nursing students, and obstetricians to the classes, where they can become involved in helping to meet parent needs and can answer parent questions about medical care and hospitals.

The Obstetrician

The attitudes of obstetricians toward childbirth education vary, ranging from outright opposition to warm support of preparation for childbirth. Their feelings for or against the new childbirth are often strong. If they feel that their patients want the new childbirth, some of them become interested in learning about prepared childbirth and family-centered maternity care. For a long time the demand was very light. There were many misconceptions about "natural" childbirth and little accurate knowledge on the part of either the public or the professionals.

Most obstetricians do not participate actively in parent education classes because they have not seen teaching classes as part of their role. Teaching requires time and training. They do, however, refer patients to childbirth classes, although they usually let this initiative come from parents. They do this partly because they do not want to recommend classes to patients who expect to be "knocked out" and who have never heard of classes, and also because doctors do not always have the latest information on the availability and content of classes.

Concerns of obstetricians have centered around several questions in addition to the question about the need of prepared women for anesthesia at birth. Does prepared childbirth really reduce pain or even eliminate it entirely as some claim? Is the emotional involvement of parents in birth really necessary or is it a non-essential frill? How does it affect the obstetrician's role? Will fathers get in the way? Will they faint? Will they leave if asked? Will the patient be disappointed if she "fails"? Doctors who have had experience with helping parents to share in the birth have found that the armchair theories about possible difficulties have presented no problem in actual practice.

Some obstetricians understand better than others the role of prepared women and their husbands in the new childbirth and the reasons why parents want to be present at birth if the woman is not in pain. Other doctors are annoyed by patient interest and the questioning of maternity care practices, nor do they really want to confront the emotions of the father and mother at the time of birth. Their surgically oriented training has not prepared them for this aspect of childbirth.

The doctor is important to the prepared woman, in some ways more so than in the traditional experience, because his role includes relationships as well as procedures. He is not just receiving the baby and watching for trouble, he is also helping parents to have a positive experience. If the obstetrician does not feel entirely adequate to serve parents in this way, he can feel rejected because prepared childbirth does place the mother and father in an active role. The woman educated for childbirth keeps her adult role. Her dependence on the doctor does not result from lack of knowledge about normal childbirth, what is happening, and what to expect about standards of care. The doctor must be aware of the needs of the new family. His patient does expect more than to bring medical questions to the doctor and to present herself at the office or at the hospital when told with minimal need for information, communication, or relationship. Although the new childbirth does involve a shift in the dynamics of the doctor-patient relationship, it is a shift which can offer satisfactions to doctor and patient. As before, the medical skills are used when needed.

Who Teaches Childbirth Education

Childbirth education teachers need special training whether or not they have a medical background. The instructor is most often a nurse with special training for prepared childbirth. Occasionally her basic preparation is in physical therapy, biology, social work, public health, or medicine.

At times a lay teacher with special training does the job. Lay teachers can be used because the preparation is for a normal birth. No pathology is taught. Because the obstetrician is in charge of the medical management of each class student, the instructor is not needed for her medical skills. Also, a lay teacher who has herself learned about and experienced childbirth can be reassuring to students. Then, too, the medical and non-medical roles are less likely to be confused. The couples in class are students, not patients. The teacher is offering education to parents.

Some teaching experience in the instructor's background is useful before she starts teaching parents about childbirth. Many people think that sensitivity training of some kind in her background is useful. The instructor should have read the available literature on childbirth education and should be aware of relevant research related to education for childbirth. She should also have attended series of classes given by different instructors, and have attended and continue to attend workshops and meetings on education for childbirth and maternity care.

There is some disagreement as to whether or not the instructor should herself be a mother. For most teachers it is an advantage to have experienced the prepared childbirth experience which she is teaching, and her students will certainly ask her what it was like for her. Most childbirth educators feel that it is important that she be a mother who has experienced prepared childbirth, but there are individuals who are not parents who have special empathy and ability to relate to others, and who have had extensive experience of a kind that gives them an understanding of parent needs. Some of the leaders in the childbirth education field have been obstetricians, nurses, and nurse-midwives with these special qualities.

The ability of an instructor to give several sides to a question is important, but couples will find that classes do present a definite point of view. The approach is not neutral or impersonal. It supports the entitlement of parents to knowledge about childbirth and it gives parents confidence that they can have a childbirth experience they will be glad to remember. The instructor's job is to teach them how.

The instructor must also be able to relate to class members in a friendly and receptive way. This quality is important in other types of teaching, too, but is especially necessary as couples prepare to have their babies and to enter a new life stage. It helps to overcome some of the inevitable depersonalization of the hospital setting.

A male figure along with the female instructor in a team teaching arrangement is often mentioned as being desirable when teaching couples. This has been tried, although infrequently. The man has been the instructor's husband, or a professional or lay father who has experienced classes and prepared childbirth. He can talk with fathers about their feelings related to childbirth and fatherhood.

Factual knowledge, healthy attitudes, the ability to relate well to students are all important to a childbirth education instructor. Her personal qualifications are every bit as important as her professional qualifications, if not more so.

Learning about Childbirth in Class

Everyone knows by now that something more is required by women than being told not to be afraid, that fear and struggle will make labor and delivery harder for them and their babies. Women have to know what childbirth is all about and how to respond to the forces within them.

Childbirth education, as a health education adjunct to medical care, offers the opportunity to promote physical and mental health at a time when people are especially receptive to change and growth. Conscious, shared childbirth is presented in classes as an experience which there is no need to try to avoid for couples who have had adequate training. The education is all directed toward (1) imparting an understanding and respect for the body and its functioning and (2) giving couples confidence in their ability to help themselves during childbirth.

When information is given women usually desire to experience birth more fully even if they had not thought about this before or known that a participating experience was possible. They find that they do desire to be present psychologically as well as physically.

The father's role—both his presence and what he can do to increase his wife's comfort in labor—is presented as important. Men are often uncertain at first about coming to class, but not as much so now that less separation is seen between men's work and women's work, with the emphasis placed on becoming more complete human beings who care. Husbands were formerly taught of their uselessness at this time in a woman's life. They may be biologically useless, but they are not psychologically useless, and it has been said that it is rather a matter of chance that the woman, not the man, carries their developing baby.

The new approach to childbirth helps to give men a way to make the transition to parenthood and to help them know what is going on with their wives. There is less rejection of the father at a critical time, and both husband and wife feel less isolated if there is a shared understanding of pregnancy and birth.

The man has a chance to develop the supportive side of himself, and during labor he will have the satisfaction of seeing that he can help to make his wife more comfortable. Usually it is not thought desirable for unprepared husbands who have not been to class to be present at labor and delivery. However, there is no advantage in being trained medically because that is not the purpose of his presence. Medical students and doctors find that they need to attend class to learn how to give husbandly support during labor. Sometimes men come to the class to learn the art of giving the coaching during labor. They then find that they like the shared communication with their wives and other couples. They also get their own doubts and questions answered in an informal setting.

When couples come to class late in pregnancy, as they

have since the advent of the Lamaze method, some women do not have time for all of the class sessions before they deliver their babies. They come late in pregnancy because they do not always find a class earlier and also because Lamaze preparation originated as a method of psychological conditioning of women. Class attendance late in pregnancy allows the conditioning, or learning, to be fresh in their minds for delivery. There are disadvantages as well as advantages to coming in the last three months of pregnancy. Expectant parents do not always have time to integrate all the information which is given to them and to make choices about the maternity care they desire. Sometimes, too, they need support during early pregnancy when they feel uncertain about many things, only some of which are brought up in the doctor's office. The suggestion is sometimes made that one or two sessions could be attended during early pregnancy to allow couples to do some reading and thinking, and also to get some reassurance about birth. The remainder of the sessions could be attended later in pregnancy so that the techniques would be fresh in their minds for birth. Some couples do come to class early and then come back later for a review session before they have their babies.

Content of Classes

Eight sessions are required to give all of the childbirth education material considered important to couples expecting a baby. A less complete course, focusing almost entirely on the labor and delivery, is frequently given and requires five or six sessions.

Although each birth is fundamentally the same, no experience is an exact duplicate of another. Students learn to accept the range of normal variations.

The outline of what is taught in an eight-session childbirth class would include the following information. Couples learn about labor and delivery, including anatomy, physiology, comfort measures, exercises, and breathing techniques. At the same time they learn about hospital procedures which are associated with labor and delivery. The importance of maintaining the muscle tone of the pelvic floor and the need for learning to relax the perineal musculature are stressed. Medication and anesthesia are discussed. Other topics are pregnancy, fetal development, postpartum and newborn care including family planning and breast feeding. The transition to parenthood is a topic which runs, directly and indirectly, throughout the course.

Instructors usually prefer either a modified Read approach or the Lamaze method, depending on their own personalities, experience, and training. They may use the Erna Wright method, another method based on psychoprophylaxis like Lamaze, or they may give a class based on the body awareness teaching of Sheila Kitzinger. All methods will work if they are well taught because of the essential ingredients which they have in common. As the modified Read classes and the Lamaze classes have changed and combined their techniques, many classes for prepared childbirth may be called Lamaze classes, so that the terms "prepared childbirth" and "Lamaze childbirth" tend to become synonymous.

A childbirth class is not a lecture class or an exercise class. Preparation is informational, physical, and attitudinal because birth is a physical and muscular event as well as an emotional event. The methods of teaching include lecture, discussion, visual aids, exercises, and rehearsals for labor and delivery combined into a unique blend which is very effective in serving its purposes.

The rehearsals for labor which are included in all childbirth classes help to integrate an awareness of body sensations with the information given and they provide an unusual opportunity to learn to work with the body. The use of touch is included in the teaching. This "laying on of hands" has tended to become a lost art but is very important in preparing women for childbirth and in supporting them during childbirth. The instructor shows the husband how to help his wife by using this supportive kind of touch. The woman gets reassurance, confidence, and an increased ability to release tense muscles. Touch also helps her to become aware of tension spots. The comfort measures, such as back rubs and abdominal lifting, and the ways of checking muscle relaxation as described in Chapter II are important.

Class Discussions

Family-based classes are challenging and rewarding experiences for both instructors and students. Expectant parents are surprisingly open in their feelings, responses, and aspirations when they come to class. They are eager for information, much more so than in the average adult education class.

At first, if class members, especially fathers, are unsure how to respond to the opportunity for discussion, instructors often toss out questions to the group. An experienced mother may be asked how she would describe what a labor contraction feels like. An experienced father may be asked what it was like to bring the baby home. The group may be asked how many are planning to breast-feed. How do those in the group feel about breast feeding? There are advantages to having first-time parents and experienced parents in the same class.

The instructor actively brings up questions for discussion and lets some answers come from the group, but she does not use the group in a way which interferes with the giving of information needed by parents from her. If the instructor is uncertain about answers to questions from the group she will say so. Absolute answers to some questions are not available. Some questions from the group are specifically obstetrical in nature, perhaps relating to pathology or individual problems. These questions belong in the obstetrician's office.

Expectant parents do have some anxiety about childbirth. All of them do. The instructor will deal openly and honestly with feelings couples have about birth but does not dig out deep fears. Classes are not the place to do this. She will talk with those who have extreme fears on an individual basis and can even refer them for special help if they wish. The better childbirth education associations usually have on their boards at least one psychiatric consultant who has an understanding of childbirth. Whatever their earlier exposure to negative or harmful influences, men and women are offered a positive experience by classes.

At the first class all those attending, including the instructor, introduce themselves, taking about a minute or so to give whatever information about themselves they wish. These introductions are possible when the classes are limited in size. Those who have had babies may say something about previous labors. Others may say why they came to class and what they hope to gain from it.

Discussions may occur during the latter part of the class session after the lecture and exercises or at any time during it when someone brings up a question. The instructor keeps enough control over the discussion so that the class does not become disorganized. The discussion should not be irrelevant to the purposes of the class or take the place of factual information and rehearsal.

When a couple and baby from a previous class series comes back to visit, students in class ask what it was like to give birth and be in the hospital, and what it is like to take care of a new baby. The questions are apt to be very searching and detailed. When asked about prepared childbirth, the initial and immediate response of the new mother is very likely to be, "It works!" She then goes on to tell what it was like the day that her baby was born.

How a Childbirth Class Is Organized

Classes are usually kept small enough to promote some individual relationship with instructors and to promote relationships among couples. Some teachers do teach large classes successfully if they are divided into small groups for part of the session.

Women are asked to wear slacks or leotards, and to bring pillows for labor rehearsals. They usually bring a permission slip from the doctor in case he does not want his patient to exercise. Doctors almost never refuse to give permission for classes. The permission slip is also a way of informing the doctor that his patient has enrolled for classes.

At the first session registration cards are usually filled out by the couples attending the class. The card usually requests name, address, telephone number, due date, name of doctor, name of hospital, ages of other children if any, and any special interest or professional background. If there is something special that students wish covered in the class they may indicate it on the card. The information helps the instructor become acquainted with the class members and may have some effect on how she presents the class. However, it has been found by instructors that whether the class is made up mostly of professional people, including doctors and nurses, or whether it is made up of students with different educational backgrounds, essentially the same information is needed by all.

If the doctor's name on the card is that of a new one who has not previously referred patients to a class, the instructor may contact him or send him some literature. If the instructor feels it necessary to speak with a doctor about an individual student, she will inform the student, but students generally do their own communicating with their doctors.

Classes usually have an assistant who helps with registration and in other ways such as procuring films, setting up chairs or moving them during exercises and labor rehearsals. The assistant helps with discussion and moves around among the couples during practice sessions, helping the instructor to check techniques. She may be a nurse from the hospital if the class is held at a hospital or a candidate in training to be a childbirth education instructor, or she may be a lay assistant who was a former class member.

The instructor may arrange for a hospital tour for the class or she will encourage students to tour the hospital in which they plan to have their babies. A tour helps to remove the mystery about what happens in the hospital and reduces anxiety about the unknown. Expectant parents inspect the equipment, ask questions, and admire the babies in the nursery.

Near the end of the series of classes the instructor passes out sheets of paper usually called labor guides or technique reminder sheets. Each instructor develops her own for use in her classes. The purpose of the guides is to remind couples what to do at each stage of labor, what is happening, and how they may feel. Couples take this guide to the hospital and they may show it to the hospital nurse to inform her what they have been taught.

Before the end of the series the instructor also passes out questionnaires to be returned to her after the baby is born. These are for the instructor's interest and for the benefit of future students. Questions are asked about what was most helpful in class for the birth, what was least helpful during labor and delivery of the information given them in class, whether mothers are breast feeding and whether they have had any difficulty with breast feeding. Besides asking for information about birth experience, couples are asked if the class gave them what they came for, whether there was anything not covered which they would like to have had covered, and asking for suggestions for future classes.

Information on community resources may be given, such as the availability of labor coaches or monitrices, or information on how to reach nursing mothers groups for assistance with breast feeding.

After the delivery, couples often get together once more for a reunion. At times the benefits have been beyond price in preventing difficulties for a new family. Nowhere else can they get the benefits of a group experience with other new parents under the guidance of an informed instructor.

The value often goes far beyond that of a social occasion which brings couples together once more, this time with their babies. They compare notes on birth, medical care, and child care. They sort out the advice given to them and discuss the life styles they are choosing or have chosen.

Teaching Aids

Teaching aids are only aids and not substitutes for the other ingredients of the class. They can be useful and interesting to class members. The International Childbirth Education Association and the Maternity Center Association are two sources of teaching aids. They are also knowledgeable about other teaching aids which are available from other groups or institutions. Community childbirth education groups keep informed about teaching aids which are useful in childbirth classes and also produce some of their own.

Books

The International Childbirth Education Association[3] publishes a book list for parents which is often distributed to class members. Classes also provide a library of books on a table which couples can borrow. If there is a shortage of copies, students often buy books to have on hand to read at their leisure.

Charts

The Maternity Center Birth Atlas[4] containing the Dickinson-Belskie charts is used almost universally in every childbirth education class. These are photographs of exquisitely detailed sculptured models illustrating the progress of labor. They are large enough to be seen fairly adequately by a group, but students usually examine them in detail after class and read the commentary on the back of each chart.

Models

The instructor may have a model of a pelvis showing the bony structure. She illustrates the descent of the baby's head with a doll. Other teachers do not like to show the skeletal structure in this way and prefer to use charts for this demonstration. Another type of model is used to show how the cervix dilates. In this demonstration a doll is eased through the neck of a turtleneck sweater or through the outlet of a knitted sock. The use of a sock demonstrates the angle of the uterus as it joins the vagina, the foot part illustrating the uterus. A knitted uterus made with directions from the Maternity Center may be used to show the muscular action of the uterus and the dilated cervix. The models show the activity which is going on during labor and delivery, and they help to show why it is important to relax and the need to assume the semi-propped body position for delivery instead of lying flat.

Films

Parents usually see one or two films on birth during a series of classes. Sometimes a film about breast feeding is shown. The time spent on film showings is limited because if films are overused they are not worth the time spent. There is no ideal film which covers all of the important teaching points, or one which may not give misconceptions or distortions to viewers. Scenes which may give an incorrect impression have to be explained in advance and discussed after the film is shown. A film guide[5] is published by the International Childbirth Education Association which is revised periodically as new films continue to be produced.

Films give a visual experience of birth which helps misconceptions to be replaced by the reality of what happens during birth. They also open up questions for discussion. A good film for parents emphasizes how the mother makes herself more comfortable and how she is helped by those around her. The faces of the mother, father, and baby are much more important than any medical procedures shown. How the people are feeling and responding to the event of birth is most important. There is no purpose in watching an inert and unconscious woman being delivered.

Couples are prepared ahead of time for the head-on perineal view of birth by learning about birth and seeing the charts and models. Even so, the visual experience of watching a woman give birth does have a strong impact on viewers, although they are not necessarily made uncomfortable. However, any blood often looks extra red even if the quantity is small. The newborn may look extra blue. Viewers may have feelings of being overwhelmed by the birth, especially when the baby emerges, makes his first cry, and is given to his parents.

Choosing a Class

Parents, nurses, and doctors need ways of evaluating a class without the necessity of attending all of the sessions. There is no real substitute for attending the class, but parents seeking a class want to know how to choose one. Hospitals and parent groups that wish to train and hire childbirth education instructors want guidelines. Many people have not known what a high-quality class should include.

Just as certain questions must be asked when selecting an obstetrician and hospital, the class instructor must be asked certain questions. The couples who are looking for a class usually telephone her or perhaps call a registrar in charge of classes if classes are sponsored by a community group. Brochures about classes are usually available.

Couples must first decide whether they desire a five- or six-session class which will focus almost entirely on the labor and delivery, or whether they want an eight-session class which will include other topics such as pregnancy, breast feeding, recovery from childbirth, maternity care practices, care of the new baby, and contraception. The eight-session class will also probably offer more than one film and an opportunity for class discussion not often available in a five- or six-session class, at least not to the same extent.

Couples must also decide, if there is a choice, whether they have strong feelings on which method of prepared childbirth they wish to learn. Some people feel more secure in an authoritarian, drill-type class which is very specific at all times. Others prefer a more flexible, body-awareness type of approach.

Prospective students might want to know who sponsors the classes and whether the instructor's attitudes are similar to theirs. Does she feel that people in her classes usually do well with prepared childbirth? They will want to know how large the class is and whether the instructor has an assistant. What exercises and breathing techniques are taught? What topics are covered? They should also ask how much time, approximately, is spent on lecture, on discussion, and on rehearsal. They will perhaps want to know what records are kept. Are the records available (anonymous and coded) to class students who want to read about the prepared childbirth experience as described by parents who were former students in the class? Is there any other follow-up after the classes such as an opportunity for a class reunion or help with breast feeding? Students might want to know what teaching aids are used. A library of books which are available for borrowing is very important in a childbirth education class.

A Final Word

Most people have been isolated from accurate knowledge about childbirth and from the issues involved in maternity care even though everyone's life is touched in some way by the ways in which childbirth is handled. The public has not felt entitled to knowledge, or cared to know, because childbirth was thought to be too painful, too medical, and too unpleasant to know about. Childbirth classes which give training for a conscious, shared experience cannot help but give at the same time an opportunity to know about birth and maternity care practices.

The new childbirth learned in class is a physiological kind of childbirth as opposed to childbirth largely controlled by the wonders of technology. Technology is important, even life-saving at times. Because it can effect such dramatic results, it becomes tempting to overuse it, but if technological interference is used routinely for normal births as a replacement for education and personalized care it tends to create its own problems for which more technology must be devised. The long-term consequences cannot always be known. Overdependence on technology is true in areas of life other than that of maternity care where short-term expedience often takes precedence over long-term effects on human life. Perhaps some of the human elements contained in childbirth education can spread beyond the confines of maternity care to other problems of society where depersonalization and loss of dignity tend to occur. If new parents and babies are not deserving of this care, there seems less hope that it will be available elsewhere in society.

The words "safety" and "prevention" can mean different things to different people. So can the words "conservative" and "radical." For many obstetricians in the United States the goal has been a medicated, spinal-forceps delivery. This method of handling childbirth these men see as the conservative one. Others see it not as conservative but as involving a good deal of interference with physiological processes. However, this approach to childbirth did seem to make sense when there was no alternative method to use. It seemed safer. The thinking goes like this. For the untrained woman the medication removes much of the anxiety about birth and relaxes her so that she does not struggle against the birth. The spinal anesthesia insures relaxation of the perineal tissues, and the forceps give the doctor better control over the delivery. An induced labor gives protection against possible emergency childbirth in the car and is a convenience to mother and doctor. The vitamin K is a protection against possible lack of blood-clotting ability in the baby. The pitocin or other oxytocic drug speeds the labor and makes sure that the uterus clamps down after delivery. The mother's hands are strapped down to prevent harm to herself or her baby under drugs. The father's absence is safer because he might faint or become emotionally upset if he attended the birth. He might also cause infection. The baby is suctioned with a bulb-suction device in case there is mucus in his mouth and throat. There is delay in sucking and feeding opportunities for the baby because of the drugs. The baby is kept away from the mother so that she won't get tired. The episiotomy is routinely done to prevent prolapse, cystoceles, and rectoceles in later life.

This is the type of maternity care which the majority of women in the United States are receiving. It assumes that parents do not know how to cope with childbirth, and without preparation it is true that they do not know how to cope with it. Practices are changing in hospitals. Recently Massachusetts became one of the states to encourage family-centered care. The public was informed in a newspaper announcement that "The Public Health Department is encouraging hospitals to permit natural childbirth and the attendance of fathers in the labor and delivery rooms."[6]

The medical profession and parents in the Netherlands see safety and prevention in another way.[7] The Dutch have not yet allowed the physiological approach to become dominated by technology. The following facts have meaning to those who have learned about childbirth.

Although 70% of Dutch babies are still born at home with the aid of a midwife and maternity aide, it is very safe to have a baby in Holland. The Netherlands has one of the lowest infant mortality rates in the world in contrast to the United States.

Education for childbirth is available to most Dutch mothers, although many do not take advantage of it because they are accustomed to birth in the home and know about birth. There is an attempt to bring the home atmosphere to the hospital. The husband is considered an important analgesic and attends 80% of the deliveries. This figure is higher for home deliveries. In the hospital and at home parents are together with their baby for the first hour or two after birth before the mother takes a nap.

Induced labor is never undertaken unless there is definite medical indication. There is recognition, too, that induced labors may require the use of analgesic drugs. Dutch physicians recognize that routine premedicants during labor have an unpredictable effect on newborns. Scopolamine is considered a barbarous drug to use for women in labor.

Women labor and deliver in the same bed. They are therefore spared the fear, however unlikely, that they will involuntarily push out their baby before the attendants are ready to receive it. The delivery table, when it is "broken" for delivery, has no place for the baby to go but onto the floor if no one should be ready to receive it, a situation which in itself can cause tension in the mother. The mother's legs are rarely in stirrups because this procedure is considered detrimental to the mother even though convenient for nurse or doctor.

If there must be "artificial" birth, as it is called, instead of spontaneous delivery, the vacuum extractor is preferred to forceps; 2.5% of Dutch babies are born with the use of the vacuum extractor and 1.5% of babies are born with the use of forceps; 1.5% of live births are Caesarean. "Artificial" birth is considered traumatic enough to the mother to keep her in bed for three days. If she has had a normal, spontaneous birth she is allowed out of bed the same day of birth to go the bathroom.

The cord is not cut immediately. Placental transfusion is allowed to take place, a process whereby the blood in the placenta is allowed to flow into the cord before it is cut. This is considered helpful to the spontaneous expulsion of the placenta without manual or chemical assistance. It is also considered beneficial to the infant in preventing future anemia. The process is not hurried by "milking" of the cord but is allowed to take about four minutes. Abdominal pressure and massage are avoided in an effort to minimize the possibility of Rh sensitization. Vitamin K is not routinely administered unless labor is prolonged or the birth is "artificial." After delivery oxytocin is not given routinely.

Episiotomies are not routinely done either. The three reasons which are given in America have not been found valid by Dutch physicians. These are: (1) possible increase in gynecological problems; (2) extra pressure on the baby's head during delivery; and (3) diminished sexual satisfaction of husbands after the birth of the baby. However, it is important to note that the pelvic floor exercise is taught to all Dutch women.

The present way of handling childbirth in the Netherlands is an example of one different from maternity care practices as they evolved in the United States. The Dutch physician is also interested in health and safety, but his goal, and that of the nurse-midwife, is a conscious, spontaneous delivery.

It is an art to use the benefits of technology in ways

that help, that do not interfere with normal physiological processes, and that do not produce unnecessary stress for the new family. The development of more new drugs for normal childbirth could at one time be seen as progress, but this direction no longer makes sense.

There were reasons for the traditional ways of handling childbirth in the United States and these ways were long taken for granted by both the public and professionals. The public is now able to talk about maternity care and to have dialogue with maternity care workers. This progress, along with the professional rethinking of a significant number of nurses and doctors, has caused the traditional care to be re-examined to meet contemporary needs.

APPENDIX

Childbirth Education Associations
Affiliated with the ICEA* or ASPO**

In addition to the affiliated groups, there are individual members of these associations. ASPO has membership categories for instructors and physicians. There are 329 instructor members and 138 physician members. A few of the ICEA groups listed below hold individual rather than group memberships. The La Leche League as described in Chapter VI often helps couples to find childbirth classes. It also often helps them to choose a doctor or hospital interested in prepared childbirth.

Arizona
   Tucson Childbirth Education Association
   3838 Calle Fernando, Tucson 85716 (ICEA)

California
   Childbirth Education League of Monterey
   P. O. Box 6628, Carmel 93921
   (individual member ICEA)

* International Childbirth Education Association, Box 5852, Milwaukee, Wisc.
** American Society for Psycho-prophylaxis in Obstetrics, Inc., 7 W. 96th St., New York, N.Y. 10025.

Childbirth Education Association of Los Angeles
  1205 Emerald Bay, Laguna Beach 92641
  (individual member ICEA)
Merced Branch—ICEA
  2353 W. McSwaine Rd., Merced 95340
  (individual member ICEA)
Childbirth Without Pain—Prepared Parents Leagues
  3744 Comer Ave., Riverside 92507 (ICEA)
Education for Childbirth Association of San Diego
  Teresita St., San Diego 92140 (ICEA)
Department of Adult Education
  81 N. 7th St., San Jose 95112 (ICEA)
A.S.P.O. Bay Area (chapter ASPO)
  Box 5042, Elmwood Station, Berkeley 94705
A.S.P.O. Los Angeles (chapter)
  2727 Patricia Ave., Los Angeles 90064
A.S.P.O. Sacramento Valley (chapter)
  Box 4553, Sacramento 95825
San Diego CEA (ASPO affiliate)
  4308 Adams Ave., San Diego 92116

Colorado
Childbirth Education Association of the Pikes Peak Region
  1903 Cascade Lane, Colorado Springs 80906 (ICEA)
Poudre Valley Childbirth Education Association
  Box 56, Fort Collins 80521 (ICEA)
Childbirth Education Association of Pueblo
  2220 Pine, Pueblo 81004
  (individual member ICEA)

Connecticut
Parents Association for Childbirth Education
  24 Trotwood, West Hartford 06107 (ICEA) (ASPO)
Connecticut C.A.L.M.
  38 Bayberry Lane, Westport 06880 (ASPO affiliate)

Florida
Childbirth and Parent Association
7261 S.W. 9th St., Miami 33144 (ICEA)

Illinois
A.S.P.O. Chicago (chapter)
537 Butterfield Rd., Libertyville 60048
CEA of Peoria
233 Campanile, Peoria 61600 (ASPO affiliate)

Indiana
Association for Childbirth Education, Inc.
251 Wells St., Crown Point 46307 (ASPO affiliate)

Maine
Maternal-child Health Council of Greater Bangor
160 Broadway, Bangor 04401 (ICEA)

Maryland
Childbirth Education Association of Baltimore
4605 Pen Lucy Rd., Baltimore 21229 (ICEA)
Parent and Child
11405 Soward Drive, Kensington 20795 (ICEA)

Massachusetts
Childbirth Education Association of Greater Springfield
Box 38, East Longmeadow 01028 (ICEA)
Boston Association for Childbirth Education, Inc.
Box 29, Newtonville 02160 (ICEA)
Pioneer Valley CEA
Box 784, Amherst 01002 (ASPO affiliate)
Franklin County Association for Lamaze Childbirth
#4 Brookside, Greenfield 01301 (ASPO affiliate)
Childbirth Education Association of Central Massachusetts
Box 73, Worcester 01606 (ICEA)

Michigan

Lamaze Childbirth Preparation Association
2451 Tranton Court, Ann Arbor 48105
(individual member ICEA)
Lamaze Childbirth Preparation Association
P. O. Box 14, Flint 48501 (ASPO affiliate)
Childbirth Preparation Service
2659 Fairway Drive, Jackson 49201 (ASPO affiliate)

Missouri

Childbirth Education Association of Greater Kansas City
8814 Glenwood, St. Louis 64138 (ICEA)

New Jersey

Childbirth Education Association of New Jersey
251 Nottingham Way, Hillside 07205 (ICEA)
A.S.P.O. Central New Jersey
334 Carlton Club Drive, Piscataway 08854 (chapter)
A.S.P.O. Northern New Jersey
90 E. Crescent Ave., Allendale 07401 (chapter)
A.S.P.O. Princeton
72 Dempsey St., Princeton 08540 (chapter)
Childbirth Education Association of South Jersey
P. O. Box 49, Clarksboro 08020 (ICEA)

New York

CEA of Rochester
22 Nunda Blvd., Rochester 14610 (ASPO affiliate)
A.S.P.O. Buffalo
2854 Main St., Buffalo 14214 (chapter)
A.S.P.O. Long Island
301 Marlin St., Dix Hills, Deer Park P.O.,
Long Island 11729 (chapter)
A.S.P.O. New York City
7 W. 96th St., New York 10025
A.S.P.O. Southern Tier
1034 Elwood Ave., Endwell 13760

A.S.P.O. Westchester
   812 Lorena St., Mamaroneck 10543
Family Centered Maternity Association
   Box 2676, Schenectady 12309 (ASPO affiliate)
CEA of Albany
   3 Garden Terrace, Delmar 12054 (ASPO affiliate)
Childbirth Education Association of Tomkins County
   R.D. #3, Trumansburg 14886

Ohio
Childbirth Education Association of Akron
   175 Dodge Ave., Akron 44302
   (individual member ICEA)
Husband-Coached Natural Childbirth Association
   9631 Loveland-Madiera Rd., Loveland 45140 (ICEA)
Association for Parent Education
   3516 Ingleside Rd., Shaker Heights 44120 (ICEA)

Oregon
Southern Oregon Childbirth Education Association Chapter
   77 Murphy Rd., Medford 97501 (ICEA)

Pennsylvania
Pittsburgh Organization for Childbirth Education
   501 B Guys Run Rd., Cheswick 15024
   (individual member ICEA)
Childbirth Education Association of Greater Philadelphia
   P. O. Box 19101, Philadelphia 19405 (ICEA)
A.S.P.O. Philadelphia
   228 W. 67th Ave., Philadelphia 19126 (chapter)
A.S.P.O. Pittsburgh
   Box 10177, Pittsburgh 15232 (chapter)

Rhode Island
Childbirth Education Association of Rhode Island
   P. O. Box 9, North Scituate 02857 (ICEA)

Tennessee

Childbirth Education Association of Oak Ridge
P. O. Box 551, Oak Ridge 37830 (ICEA)
A.S.P.O. Nashville
513 Woodhurst Drive, Nashville 37520 (chapter)

Texas

Austin Parent-Child Association
3404 Exposition, Austin 78703
(individual member ICEA)
Dallas Association for Parent Education
7711 La Sabrina, Dallas 75240 (ICEA)

Vermont

Vermont Association for Family-Centered Care
1306 Ethan Allen Drive, Apt. 2-G, Winooski 05404
(ICEA)

Virginia

A.S.P.O. Washington, D.C.
2807 Fort Drive, Alexandria 2203 (chapter)

Washington

Childbirth Education League
P. O. Box 188, Lynwood 98036
(individual member ICEA)
Childbirth Education Association of Seattle
P. O. Box 1522, Seattle 98103 (ICEA)
Tacoma Childbirth Education Association
7925 Steilacoam Blvd., S.W. Tacoma 98498 (ICEA)

Wisconsin

Childbirth Education Association
28 Howard Ave., Fond Du Lac 54935 (ICEA)
Natural Childbirth Association of Milwaukee
11420 Belmar Drive, Hales Corner 53130 (ICEA)

Childbirth Education Services
 P. O. Box 109, Racine 53403 (ICEA)

Australia
 Childbirth and Family Life Education Association
 124 Holt Rd., Taren Point, New South Wales

NOTES

Preface

1. Doris and John Haire, *Implementing Family-Centered Maternity Care with a Central Nursery* (International Childbirth Education Association, ICEA Supplies Center, 208 Ditty Bldg., Bellevue, Wash. 98004, or Box 22, Hillside, N.J. 07205), 1971.

2. William Windle, Ph.D., Sc.D., "Brain Damage at Birth," *Journal of the American Medical Association*, Vol. 206, No. 9 (November 25, 1968).

3. *Time* magazine, May 9, 1969, p. 81.

4. David Rutstein, M.D., "Why Do We Let These Babies Die?" *Reader's Digest*, August 1964.

5. A. Towbin, M.D., Boston *Globe*, September 15, 1971 (from August 30, 1971, issue of the *Journal of the American Medical Association*).

6. Ibid., "Spinal Cord and Brain Stem Injuries at Birth," *Archives of Pathology* 77:620–632, 1964.

7. Jessie Bierman, M.D., "Some Things Learned," *American Journal of Public Health*, Vol. 59, No. 6 (June 1969), pp. 932–33.

8. Kenneth Niswander, M.D., and Robert Patterson, M.D., "Hazards of Elective Induction of Labor," *Obstetrics and Gynecology* 22:228–233, August 1963.

9. Kent Ueland, M.D., and John Hansen, M.D., "Maternal

Cardiovascular Dynamics. Posture and Uterine Contractions," *American Journal of Obstetrics and Gynecology*, Vol. 103, No. 1 (January 1969).

10. T. Berry Brazelton, M.D., "Psychophysiologic Reactions in the Neonate. Effect of Maternal Medication on the Neonate and His Behavior," *Journal of Pediatrics* 58:513–518, 1961.

11. S. Walsh, "Maternal Effects of Early and Late Clamping of the Umbilical Cord," *Lancet* 1:996–997, 1968.

12. L. Weinstein, W. Farabow, and J. Gusdon, "Third Stage of Labor and Transplacental Hemorrhage," *Obstetrics and Gynecology* 37:90–93, 1971.

13. E. Wilson, W. Windle, and H. Alt, "Deprivation of Placental Blood as Cause of Iron Deficiency in Infants," *American Journal of Diseases of Children* 62:320–327, 1941.

Chapter I

1. Robert Bradley, M.D., *Husband-Coached Childbirth* (New York: Harper & Row, 1965).

2. Erik H. Erikson, *Childhood and Society*, 2nd ed. (New York: W. W. Norton Co., 1963), pp. 420–21.

3. John Bowlby, M.D., *Child Care and the Growth of Love* (Baltimore, Md.: Pelican Books, 1953, 1965).

4. Erna Wright, *Periods without Pain* (ICEA Supplies Center, 208 Ditty Bldg., Bellevue, Wash. 98004).

5. Gertie F. Marx, M.D., and Louis R. Orkin, M.D., *Physiology of Obstetric Anesthesia* (Springfield, Ill.: Charles C. Thomas, 1969).

6. Charles E. Flowers, Jr., M.D., *Obstetric Analgesia and Anesthesia* (New York: Hoeber, medical division of Harper & Row, 1967).

7. *Husbands in the Delivery Room* (ICEA Supplies Center, 208 Ditty Bldg., Bellevue, Wash. 98004), 2nd ed., 1968.

Chapter II

1. Ruth and Edward Brecher, eds., *An Analysis of Human Sexual Response* (New York: New American Library, 1966).

2. Lester Hazell, *Commonsense Childbirth* (New York: G. P. Putnam's Sons, 1969).

3. L. Chertok, M.D., "Psychosomatic Methods of Preparation for Childbirth," *American Journal of Obstetrics and Gynecology*, Vol. 98, No. 5 (July 1, 1967), pp. 698–707.

4. Pierre Vellay, M.D., *Sex Development and Maternity*, trans. Elliot E. Philipp (London: Hutchinson & Co., 1968). Vellay, *Childbirth with Confidence* (New York: The Macmillan Co., 1969).

5. *Pain* (U. S. Dept. of Health, Education and Welfare. National Institutes of Health), September 1968.

6. Erna Wright, *The New Childbirth* (New York: Hart Publishing Co., 1966).

7. Sheila Kitzinger, *The Experience of Childbirth* (London: Victor Gollancz, Ltd., 1964; Pelican Books, 1967).

8. Edmund Jacobsen, *How to Relax and Have Your Baby* (New York: McGraw-Hill, 1959).

9. Alexander Lowen, M.D., *The Betrayal of the Body* (New York: Collier-Macmillan Co., 1969).

Chapter III

1. Gregory White, M.D., *Emergency Childbirth* (Police Training Foundation, 3412 Ruby St., Franklin Park, Ill. 60131, 2nd printing, 1968).

2. Marion Lesser and Vera Keane, *Nurse-Patient Relation-*

ship in a Hospital Maternity Service (St. Louis, Mo.: C. V. Mosby Co., 1956).

3. Madelin Alk, ed., *The Expectant Mother*, prepared by *Redbook* magazine and the American College of Obstetrics and Gynecology (New York: Trident Press, 1967), p. 132.

Chapter IV

1. T. Berry Brazelton, M.D., "What Childbirth Drugs Can Do to Your Child," *Redbook* magazine, Vol. 136, No. 4 (February 1971), p. 65.

2. J. P. Greenhill, M.D., *Analgesia and Anesthesia in Obstetrics* (Springfield, Ill.: Charles C. Thomas, 1962), p. 4.

3. W. Bowes, Y. Brackbill, E. Conway, A. Steinschneider, "The Effects of Obstetric Medication on the Fetus and Infant," Vol. 35, No. 4, monograph, Society for Research in Child Development, University of Illinois (Chicago: Chicago University Press, June 1970).

Chapter V

1. *The First Breath* (National Childbirth Trust, 41a Reeves Mews, London, W.1, England).

2. Maria Ebner, *Physiotherapy in Obstetrics* (Edinburgh and London: F. & S. Livingstone Ltd., 1967).

3. *Preparation for Childbearing* (Maternity Center Association, 48 E. 92nd St., New York, N.Y. 10028).

Chapter VI

1. The La Leche League International, Franklin Park, Ill. 60131.

2. *The Womanly Art of Breastfeeding* (Franklin Park, Ill.: La Leche League International, rev. 1963).

3. Niles Newton, *The Family Book of Child Care* (New York: Harper and Bros., 1957).

4. Haire, op. cit.

5. Ibid.

6. J. Glaser, "The Dietary Prophylaxis of Allergic Diseases in Infancy," *Journal of Asthma Research* 3:199–208, 1966.

7. Committee on Nutrition, "Report on the Feeding of Solid Foods to Infants," *Pediatrics*, Vol. 21, No. 4 (1958), pp. 685–92.

8. Brecher, op. cit., p. 90.

Chapter VII

1. Hon, Edward, *An Introduction to Fetal Heart Monitoring* (Corometrics Medical Systems, Inc., North Haven, Conn.).

2. Williams and Richards, "Fetal Monitoring," *American Journal of Nursing*, November 1970, p. 2388.

3. ICEA Supplies Center, 208 Ditty Bldg., Bellevue, Wash. 98004.

4. Maternity Center Association, 48 E. 92nd St., New York, N.Y. 10028.

5. *Directory of Films and Records*, rev. by Abigail Avery, 4th ed. (ICEA Supplies Center).

6. Boston *Globe*, January 13, 1971.

7. *ICEA News*, Vol. 9, No. 2 (November–December 1970).

BIBLIOGRAPHY

1. Bierman, Jessie, M.D. "Some Things Learned," *American Journal of Public Health*, Vol. 59, No. 6 (June 1969), pp. 932–33.

2. Bing, Elisabeth. *Six Practical Lessons for Easier Childbirth*. New York: Grosset and Dunlap, 1967.

3. Bowes, W., Brackbill, Y., Conway, E., Steinschneider, A. "The Effects of Obstetric Medication on the Fetus and Infant," Vol. 35, No. 4, monograph, Society for Research in Child Development, 1341 Euclid St., University of Illinois. Chicago: Chicago University Press, June 1970.

4. Bowlby, John, M.D. *Child Care and the Growth of Love*, 2nd ed. Baltimore, Md.: Pelican Books, 1965.

5. Bradley, Robert, M.D. *Husband-Coached Childbirth*. New York: Harper & Row, 1965.

6. Brazelton, T. Berry, M.D. "Psychophysiologic Reactions in the Neonate. Effects of Maternal Medication on the Neonate and His Behavior," *Journal of Pediatrics* 58:513–518, 1961.

7. Brecher, Ruth, and Brecher, Edward, eds. *An Analysis of Human Sexual Response*. New York: New American Library, 1966.

8. Chabon, I., M.D. *Awake and Aware*. New York: Delacorte Press, 1966.

9. Chertok, L., M.D. *Motherhood and Personality: Psychosomatic Aspects of Childbirth*. Philadelphia and New York: J. B. Lippincott, 1969.

10. Chertok, L., M.D. "Psychosomatic Methods of Preparation for Childbirth," *American Journal of Obstetrics and Gynecology*, Vol. 98, No. 5 (July 1, 1967), pp. 698–707.

11. Ebner, Maria. *Physiotherapy in Obstetrics*. Edinburgh and London: F. & S. Livingstone Ltd., 1967.

12. Erikson, Erik H. *Childhood and Society*, 2nd ed. New York: W. W. Norton Co., 1963.

13. Flowers, Charles E. Jr. *Obstetric Analgesia and Anesthesia*. New York: Hoeber (medical division, Harper & Row), 1967.

14. Glaser, J. "The Dietary Prophylaxis of Allergic Diseases in Infancy," *Journal of Asthma Research* 3:199–208, 1966.

15. Goodrich, Frederick W., M.D. *Preparing for Childbirth*. Englewood, N.J.: Prentice-Hall, Inc., 1966.

16. Gordon, R. E., M.D., and Gordon, Katherine. "Social Factors in Postpartum Problems," *Obstetrics and Gynecology* 15:433–438, 1960.

17. Haire, Doris, and Haire, John. *Implementing Family-Centered Maternity Care with a Central Nursery*. International Childbirth Education Association Education Committee, Box 22, Hillside, N.J. 07205, 1971.

18. Hazell, Lester. *Commonsense Childbirth*. New York: G. P. Putnam's Sons, 1969.

19. Karmel, Marjorie. *Thank You, Doctor Lamaze*. Philadelphia and New York: J. B. Lippincott Co., 1959.

20. Keettel, W., Randall, J., and Donnelly, M. "The Hazards of Elective Induction of Labor," *American Journal of Obstetrics and Gynecology* 75:496–510, 1958.

21. Kitzinger, Sheila. *The Experience of Childbirth*. London: Victor Gollancz Ltd., 1964.

22. Kron, R., Stein, M., Goddard, K. "Newborn Sucking Behavior Affected by Obstetrical Sedation," *Pediatrics* 37: 1012–1016, 1966.

23. Larsen, Virginia, M.D. "Stresses of the Childbearing Year," *American Journal of Public Health* 56:32–36, 1966.

24. Lowen, Alexander, M.D. *The Betrayal of the Body*. New York: Collier-Macmillan Co., 1969.

25. Marx, Gertie, M.D., and Orkin, L., M.D. *Physiology of Obstetric Anesthesia*. Springfield, Ill.: Charles C. Thomas, 1969.

26. Miller, H. Lloyd. "Education for Childbirth," *Obstetrics and Gynecology*, Vol. 17, No. 11 (January 1961).

27. Miller, John S., M.D. *Childbirth, A Manual for Pregnancy and Delivery*. New York: Atheneum, 1963.

28. Morris, Marian. "Psychological Miscarriage: An End to Mother Love," *Transaction*, January–February 1966.

29. Moss, A., and Monset-Couchard, M. "Placental Transfusion: Early versus Late Clamping of the Umbilical Cord," *Pediatrics* 40:109–126, 1967.

30. Newton, N., and Newton, M., M.D. "The Propped Position for the Second Stage of Labor," *Obstetrics and Gynecology* 15:28–34, 1960.

31. Niswander, K., and Patterson, R. "Hazards of Elective Induction," *Obstetrics and Gynecology* 22:228–233, 1963.

32. Read, Grantly Dick-. *Childbirth without Fear*. New York: Harper & Row, 1959.

33. *Standards for Obstetric-Gynecologic Hospital Services*. American College of Obstetricians and Gynecologists, 79 W. Monroe St., Chicago, Ill. 60603, 1969.

34. Tanzer, Deborah. "Natural Childbirth: Pain or Peak Experience," *Psychology Today*, October 1968.

35. *Time* magazine, May 9, 1969, p. 81.

36. Towbin, A., M.D. "Spinal Cord and Brain Stem Injuries at Birth," *Achives of Pathology* 77:620–632, 1964.

37. Ueland, Kent, M.D., Hansen, John, M.D. "Maternal Cardiovascular Dynamics. Posture and Uterine Contractions," *American Journal of Obstetrics and Gynecology*, Vol. 103, No. 1 (January 1969), pp. 1–7.

38. Vellay, Pierre, M.D. *Childbirth with Confidence*. New York: The Macmillan Co., 1969.

39. Windle, William, Ph.D. "Brain Damage at Birth," *Journal of the American Medical Association*, Vol. 206, No. 9 (November 25, 1968).

40. *Womanly Art of Breast Feeding*. Franklin Park, Ill.: La Leche League International.

41. Wright, Erna. *The New Childbirth*. New York: Hart Publishing Co., 1966.

42. Yahia, Clement, M.D., and Ulin, Priscilla, RN, M.N.

"Preliminary Experience with a Psychophysical Program of Preparation for Childbirth," *American Journal of Obstetrics and Gynecology*, Vol. 93, No. 7 (December 1, 1965), pp. 942–49.